A Simple Introduction to CBT: Wha
Behaviour Therapy is and how it wc
worksheets, and advice about key C

Dr James Manning, ClinPsyD
Dr Nicola Ridgeway, ClinPsyD

A product of the West Suffolk CBT Service Ltd, Angel Corner, 8 Angel Hill, Bury St Edmunds, Suffolk, IP33 1UZ

This edition printed 2016
Copyright (c) 2016 West Suffolk CBT Service Ltd

All rights reserved. No part of this publication may be reproduced, stored in a retrieval system, or transmitted in any form or by any means, electronic, mechanical, photocopying, recording, scanning, or otherwise, except as permitted under copyright legislation, without the prior permission of the West Suffolk CBT Service Ltd. Limits of liability/disclaimer of warranty –

Neither the authors nor the West Suffolk CBT Service Ltd take responsibility for any possible consequences from any treatment, procedure, test exercise or action of any person reading or following the information in this book. The publication of this book does not constitute the practice of medicine and this book does not attempt to replace any other instructions from your doctor or qualified practitioner. The authors and the West Suffolk CBT Service advise the reader to check with a doctor or qualified practitioner before undertaking any course of treatment.

Whilst the authors and the West Suffolk CBT Service Ltd have used their best efforts in preparing this book, they make no representations or warranties with respect to the accuracy or the completeness of the contents of this book and specifically disclaim any implied warranties or merchantability or fitness for a particular purpose. No warranty may be created or extended. The advice and strategies contained herin may not be suitable for your situation. You should where necessary consult with a professional where appropriate.

Neither the West Suffolk CBT Service or the authors shall be liable for any loss or profit or any other commercial damages, including but not limited to special, incidental, consequential or other damages.

Case examples referred to in this book are generic and based on collective presentations. No relation to any specific person is either implied or intended.

About the authors

Dr Nicola Ridgeway is a Consultant Clinical Psychologist and an accredited cognitive and behavioural therapist. She lectures on cognitive behaviour therapy at the University of East Anglia, Suffolk, England, and is Clinical Director of the West Suffolk CBT Service Ltd. Together with Dr James Manning she has co-authored several books on CBT.

Dr James Manning is a Consultant Clinical Psychologist and the Managing Director of the West Suffolk CBT Service. James has post-graduate qualifications in both Clinical Psychology and Counselling Psychology. He regularly offers workshops and training to clinicians throughout the United Kingdom on Cognitive Behaviour Therapy and continues to work as a practicing therapist.

By the Authors

Think About Your Thinking to Stop Depression: A Fast and Simple System to Reduce Distress.

How to Help Your Loved One Overcome Depression

Think About Your Thinking – Cognitive Behaviour Therapy Program for depression

CBT for Panic Attacks: Simple explanations about the causes of anxiety, panic attacks and panic disorder with advice on how to stop panic symptoms using CBT

The Little Book on CBT for Depression: Simple explanations about the causes of depression, dysthymia and low mood with advice on how to stop symptoms

Cognitive Behaviour Therapy for Social Anxiety and Shyness: Simple CBT explanations for teenagers about the causes of social anxiety and shyness, including a CBT workbook to reduce anxiety and feel more relaxed in social environments.

An Introduction to Cognitive Behaviour Therapy for visual learners.

My CBT Diary

CBT Worksheets

The Big CBT Workbook

The CBT Workbook for Anxiety

The CBT Workbook for Social Anxiety

Prologue with Dr James Manning

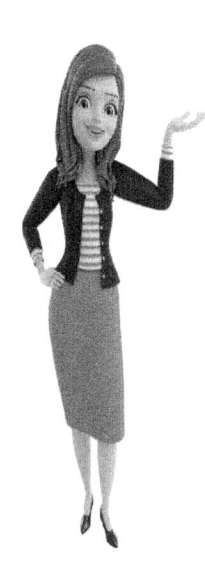

"Hi I'm Sally Blanket a Cognitive Behaviour Therapist, your guide throughout this book. Before we start talking about CBT, I'm going to be talking with one of my colleagues, James Manning, about his experience of mental health problems. James is going to be joining us now via 'live chat.' He currently works as Consultant Clinical Psychologist, in Bury St Edmunds. He told me he was quite happy for me to share his history of mental health difficulties if others might benefit from it. We'll speak to him now."

"Welcome James. I glad you could join us."

"That's no problem. Good to meet you."

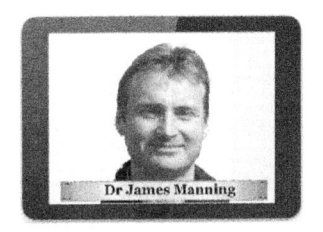

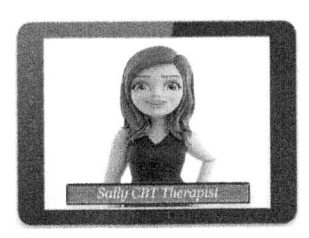

"James, as you know many people think that they're alone when they experience mental health problems. Sometimes they look around and think "What is wrong with me? Why is it that everyone else seems to be able to get on with their lives and I can't?" It would be good to hear what you have to say. I haven't heard of too many Consultant Psychologists being open about these types of issues."

"I can understand that. I think some Psychologists might think that people won't want to work with them if they've had mental health issues, or that perhaps health service managers won't employ them if they find out that they have had mental health problems."

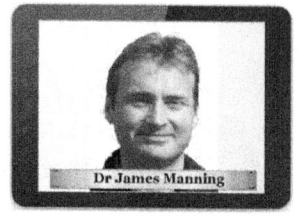

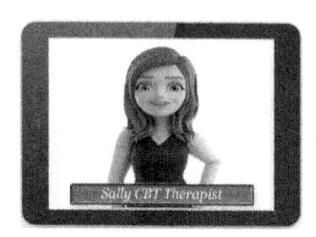

"So do you think differently?"

"Yes. I think mental health problems are very common amongst all types of professionals. Psychologists are human beings just like everyone else."

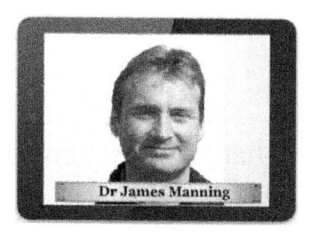

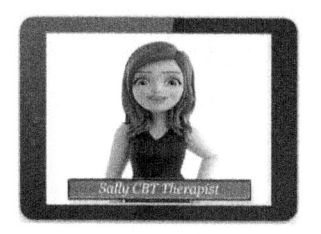

"So what happened in your life?"

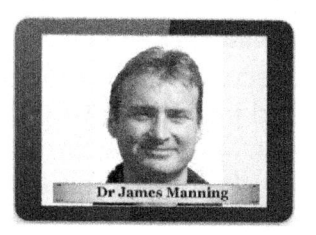

"Between the ages of 15 and 30 I experienced a type of depression, which psychiatrists would have diagnosed as dysthymia. Before this, I experienced a lot of obsessional problems and anxiety." [In dysthymia symptoms are not as intense as in major depression, but the effects of it can be experienced for a protracted period of time].

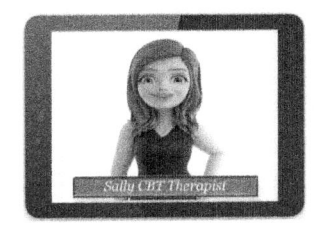

"What happened with your dysthymia?"

"I had low mood, a feeling of being slowed down, and an emptiness that sapped my motivation to engage in life. Normal events seemed more effortful and I found myself withdrawing from day to day activities. I started to feel unsettled most of the time, waking up early for no apparent reason, often at 4.00am, churning thoughts over and over in my mind and not being able to go back to sleep. I withdrew from people, preferring to be alone. I became snappy and irritable, and felt on edge most of the time. My relationships generally suffered and I lost most of my friendships."

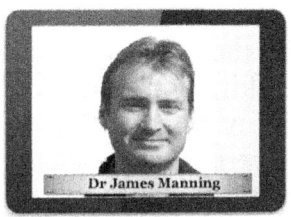

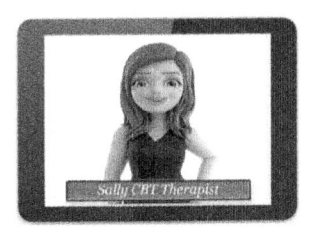

"What factors led to your dysthymia?"

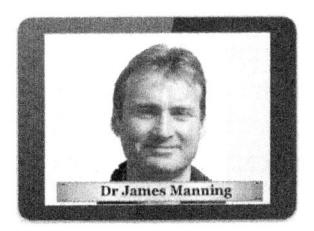

"The reasons for dysthymia are unknown. It has been suggested that dysthymia occurs as a result of physical changes in the brain, genetic factors and or environmental factors. My mother suffered from dysthymia, so I had a strong genetic pre-disposition. I also had attention deficit problems from childhood which are thought to be risk factor for future dysthymia."

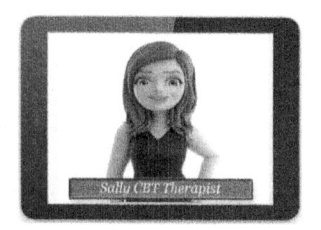

"Did anything happen in your childhood that could have contributed to it?"

"I didn't have a very eventful childhood really. Not compared to many of my clients. Both of my parents were working class people who performed well in their careers and rose through the ranks of their respective companies, in my father's case to a top management position. My father was a perfectionist and highly obsessional. His perfectionistic nature paid huge dividends for him at work financially and professionally. He supervised award winning civil engineering work. I saw an old photograph of him recently, being given an award by the Queen. He had a tendency to be obsessional in all areas, including at home, and became angry at even slight violations of his high standards. Let's say as a hormonal teenager I violated his standards pretty much all the time and he struggled with parenting me as a teenager."

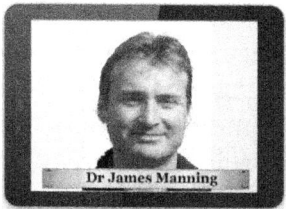

"Both my parents emigrated from Ireland at a very early age. They were very young when thrust into the responsibilities of parenthood and as you might expect from young parents they didn't really have much experience in looking after children, but they were really no different to my friends parents."

8

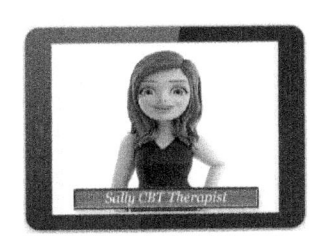

"What do you remember most about your childhood?"

"I think my parents did their best to bring me up, but I struggled with being a child. I can still hear my mother's words that she used to repeat almost daily in her soft Irish accent. "Childhood are the best years of your life, enjoy it while you can!" This confused me as my childhood felt terrible, and it seemed like my life was going to get even worse if these were the best years of my life. I had low self-esteem, and deeply entrenched beliefs that I was inadequate, stupid, bad, weak and worthless as a person. I kept these fears to myself and spent a lot of his time fighting my beliefs and trying to prove them wrong."

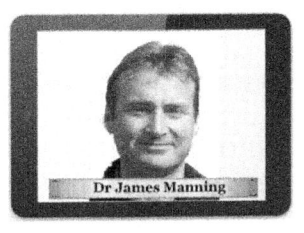

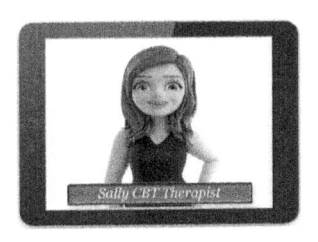

"Did you have any positive things in your life that could have helped you?"

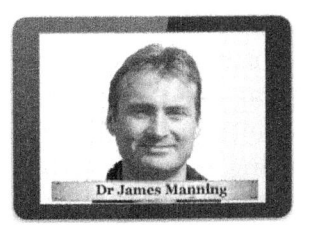

"Yes. There were a number of positives that I could have drawn something from. By the time I reached 15, outsiders would have considered me to be a privileged child. I was reasonably popular with my peers. I had the support of well off family. I lived in a leafy suburb just outside London, and attended a state selective grammar school, which at the time was one of the top schools in the country."

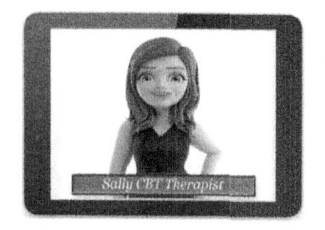

"I can see the benefits of your early life? So what went wrong?"

"Unfortunately, I was not able to use what I had been given. By the age of 15 depression had started to hit me and my motivation to engage in life had started to drop significantly. School teachers were not impressed with my academic performance and reported back to my parents that I was under-achieving academically. I passed my first set of exams at 16 and went on to do advanced exams where I achieved less than spectacular results. By the time I was doing my advanced exams teachers had noticed changes in my behaviour and had begun to monitor me more closely. One day my chemistry teacher approached me looking more perplexed than he normally did and muttered "If you're not paranoid you should be!" A short time later I was told that the teachers had had a meeting just about me and I was placed on report. This is where teachers monitor a student much more closely and have regular meetings with them. By then I had dropped out of most of my sports teams such as rugby and cross-country. I struggled with my friendship groups and eventually found myself dropped from them. Things weren't really going too well from a teenager's point of view. By this time I already felt that I was a failure in life."

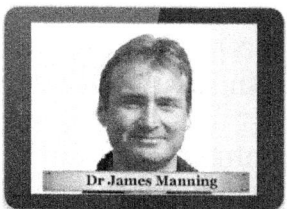

10

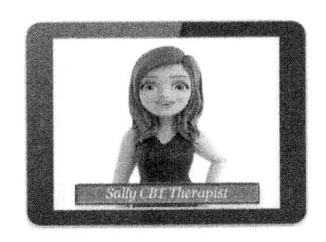

"I'm sorry to hear that you felt that way. What happened next?"

"After leaving school you could say that I had a lucky break and gained a position in a small commodity brokers."

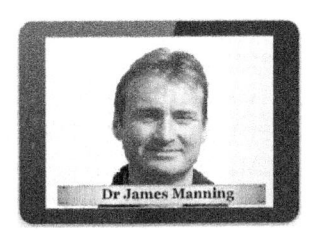

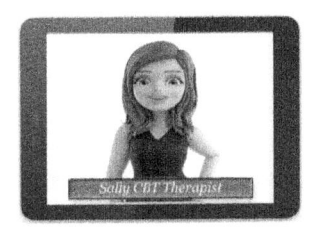

"That's sounds like a prestigious position for a young man to obtain. It must have presented you with many opportunities for career progression!"

"Yes it did. But I struggled to retain this role, not because of my mental ability, but because of my lack of ability to regulate my mood and deal with conflict. Basically, I struggled to get on with people. One day I found myself shouting at a commodity trader working for an important client. The next day I was invited to my Managing Director's office and given my notice."

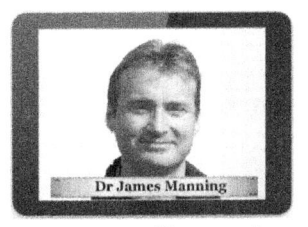

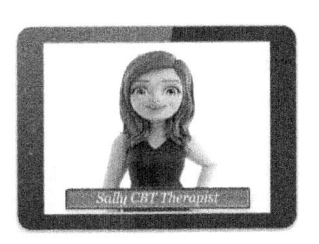

"What happened after that?"

"A number of further jobs followed, assisted at times with the support of my parents, but again I experienced interpersonal problems and had further dismissals. As time progressed I found that my CV was beginning to look less and less promising as I moved from one job to another. On paper I thought I had begun to look unemployable and started to work for financial companies with more dubious or unethical outlooks. I struggled to hold these jobs, because I could not work the way that these companies wanted me to, due to my moral stance on life. Following this, I continued to work my way down the pay scale hierarchy. Eventually the only work I could find was temporary work in factories, delivering Pizza's and working as a cleaner for a minimum wage."

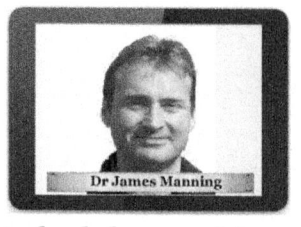

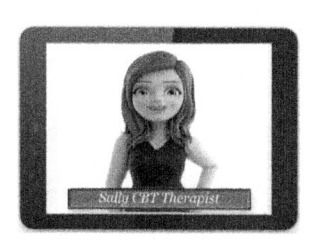

"How did you get on with these jobs? They seem very different from the jobs that you started with?"

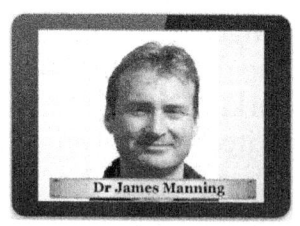

"Yes they were. Moving from plush offices to factories and such like was a bit of a culture shock. I was dismissed from two of my minimum wage cleaning jobs for not following instructions as requested. I am embarrassed to admit that the only job I didn't get the sack from before I was twenty-eight was my Pizza delivery job at Pizza Hut. Even that job was painful sometimes. From time to time I found myself delivering Pizza's to my now successful Grammar School peers who seemed shocked when they opened their door to find me standing there with a Pizza for them."

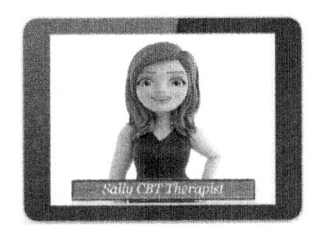

"That must have been really difficult for you?"

"Yes, it was at the time, because I had a belief that I was inadequate and what was happening to me was reinforcing it. I think by then I had switched off emotionally. During this period of time I became quite hard up financially and was quite rigid in my mind set. I didn't like to use the unemployment system or to ask my parents for help as in my mind this would have confirmed to me that I was really not succeeding in life. Sometimes I couldn't earn enough money to pay rent, so ended up for some months living in a tent at a campsite where the rent was £4 per day. At other times I could pay the rent but was left eating potatoes and baked beans as my only source of nourishment."

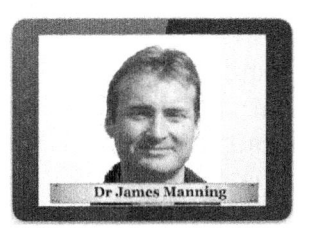

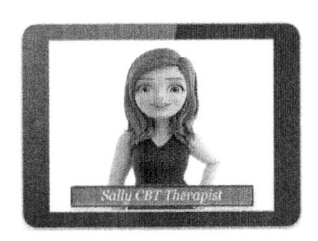

"It sounds like you hit rock bottom?"

"Yes. I continuously felt that I was failing in some way. I felt an emptiness inside. I just didn't feel like I had the energy to do things. I wanted to escape from my problems and myself. The only time I really felt OK was when I was asleep. I became quite avoidant and more nocturnal. I often did not attend events that I had been invited to, mostly without sending an apology or letting people know. I didn't answer the phone to friends or return their calls. The number of friends I had dwindled to just one. I think the only way that this friend managed to tolerate me was to laugh about the way I behaved and to recognise that my behaviour was not about him. I felt so insignificant that I genuinely believed that other people wouldn't notice or care whether I turned up late for planned events, or would even be bothered if I attended them at all. *All my focus was on myself.* I was so detached that I had little regard for other people's feelings or my own. Most of the time I felt like I didn't want to live anymore. It was as if my body, mind, and especially my personality were so unacceptable to me that I despised myself.

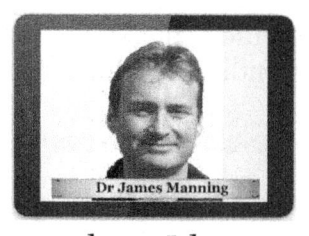

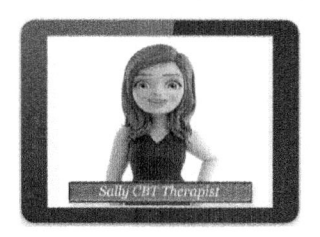

"So what happened to you in the end? You must have needed a very good therapist!"

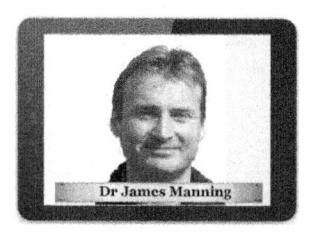

"Luckily I found a few good ones. I worked hard on my therapy, which needed a couple of years in my case, as I had left things for so long before getting help. I brought the kinds of thoughts that I had into conscious awareness and made significant changes to my life. I'm 48 now and haven't looked back since. I now try to help others who are stuck to move on with their lives."

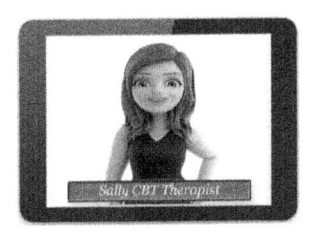

"It's good to hear that you've worked your way through your difficulties."

"Yes! I continue to use many of the exercises and coping strategies that I learnt in my therapy to keep in a good state of wellbeing."

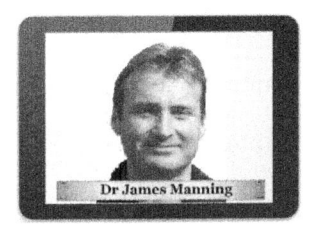

Contents

Prologue		05
Chapter 1	What happens in a CBT session	18
Chapter 2	What you will learn about the brain in early stages of therapy	25
Chapter 3	Thoughts affect the way we feel	32
Chapter 4	What makes us have distressing feelings when we think we shouldn't have them	34
Chapter 5	What causes anxiety disorders?	37
Chapter 6	What causes depression?	57
Chapter 7	Avoidance and safety behaviours	71
Chapter 8	Self-observation	83
Chapter 9	Cognitive distortions	95
Chapter 10	Rules	101
Chapter 11	Limiting beliefs	113
Chapter 12	Simple CBT cycles	130
Chapter 13	Making changes using CBT	149
Chapter 14	Challenging negative automatic thoughts	152
Chapter 15	Working with emotions	162
Chapter 16	Breaking patterns of worry and rumination	173
Chapter 17	Challenging safety behaviours	189
Chapter 18	Conclusion	215
Index		225

Regulatory Organisations	227
Glossary of terms	228
References	223
Common medications	236
Worksheets	239
Bonus Book Chapter	245

Chapter 1

What happens in a CBT session?

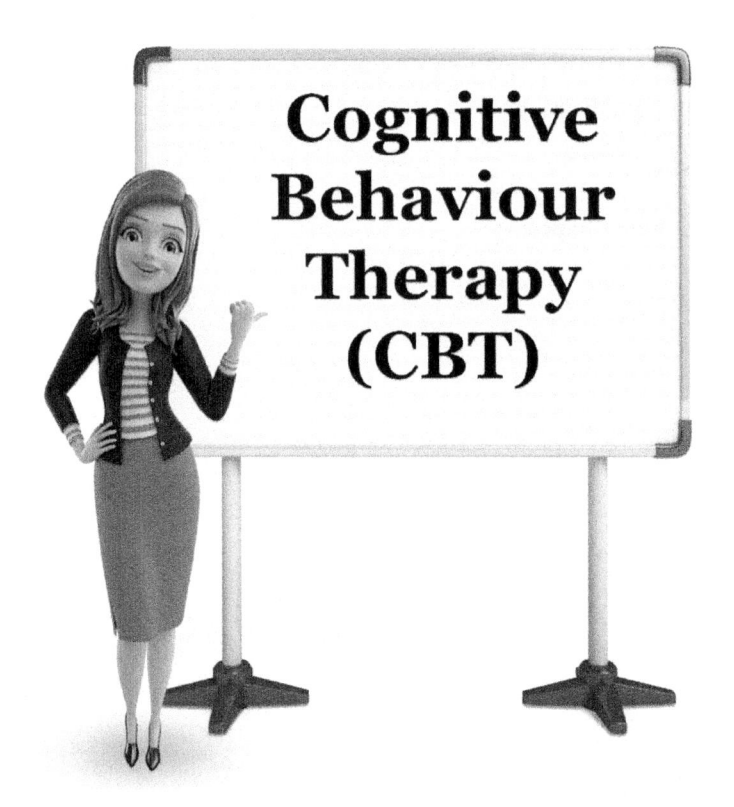

"Hi, I'm Sally Blanket a CBT practitioner. Very shortly I am going to be using 'Live Chat' to speak to our team of experts, James Smith, also known as Big Jim, Jemma Jenkins, Professor Harrold Nut, and Dr Kate Cryptic. Big Jim and Jemma have both had their own CBT in the past, Professor Knutt is an expert on the mind and Dr Kate Kryptic is a Clinical Psychologist. By the end of our chat we hope that you will know a bit more about Cognitive Behaviour Therapy, or CBT for short."

"The first guest we will be talking with today is Jemma. Jemma told me, when I asked her to be one of our guests the other day, that she experienced anxiety for as long as she could remember. She said that most of her friends didn't know that she experienced anxiety, apart from her closest friends. She had therapy after following advice from her father, who told her he had benefitted from having therapy in the past."... "Welcome Jemma, I am so grateful that you could make it."

"That's OK. I'm happy to help!"

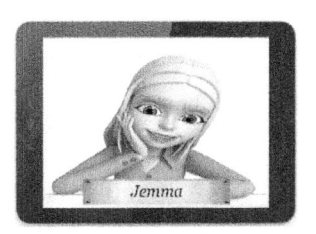

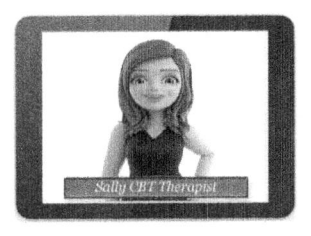

"Before we start we had better explain what cognitive behaviour therapy or CBT is for our readers. Jemma can you help our readers out by answering this question?"

"Well...Cognitive is something you do with your mind, whereas behaviour means how you act in certain situations. When people do therapy they change the way they think and behave. This helps people to feel better. People can do CBT on their own or they can do it with a therapist. I decided that I wanted to work with a therapist."

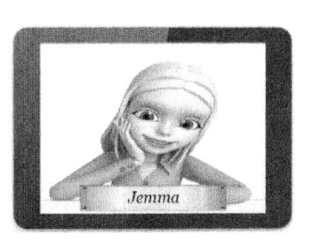

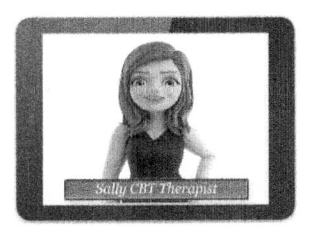

"What was it like for you going to therapy for the first time?

"My mum came with me to my first session. My therapist said it was OK for her to come in with me. After my first session I felt comfortable enough to be seen on my own so Mum waited outside in the waiting area."

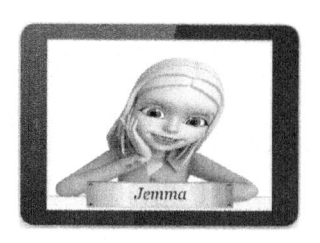

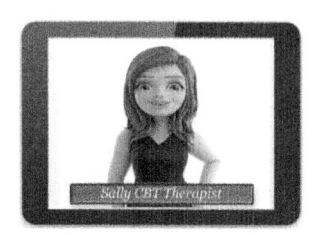

"I guess it must have been an unusual situation for you, talking to a complete stranger about some of your most difficult problems!"

"Yes it was. At first, it was something I felt really nervous about. I thought she...I mean the therapist, might judge me or something. My Dad tried to encourage me and told me all about the therapy he had in the past, so I wasn't sure what to expect. I went along for the appointment anyway because I really wanted to do something about my anxiety. I didn't know what was going to happen. After talking to Dad I thought I would have to lie down on a coach or something and be hypnotised."

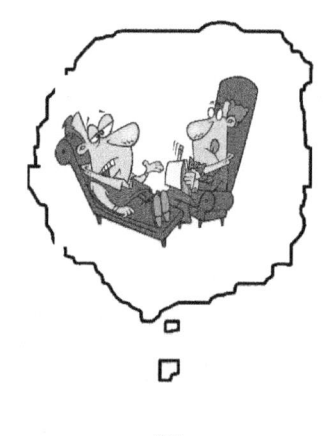

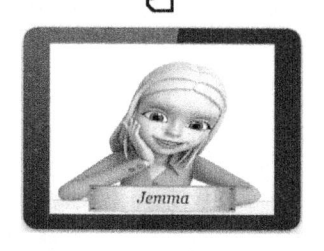

"It turned out CBT was nothing like Dad's therapy. The lady I saw seemed very normal. She asked me what my problems were. It got a bit easier once I started talking. It seemed like she understood what was happening to me. She wrote many of the things I said on a white board. By the end of my first appointment I felt I understood a lot more about myself."

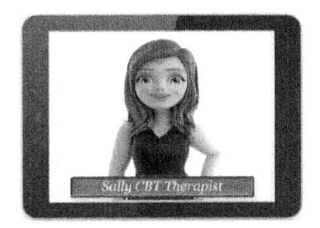

"Thank you Jemma, I think our readers will find what you have to say about CBT very interesting. I still have a lot more to ask you as we go on so if would be great if you can hang around for a bit."

"That's no problem at all!"

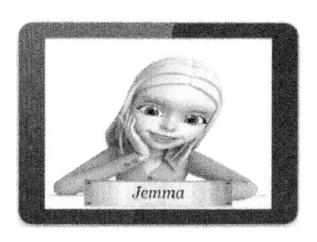

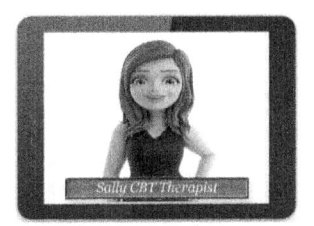

"I think for the benefit of our readers I will just explain that most CBT therapists meet with their clients on a one to one basis in their office. They know it is difficult for many people to come to their first appointment and they are usually very willing to allow relatives and other family members into the first set of meetings if you ask them."

"Like Jemma, you've also had your own therapy Big Jim. What was it like for you in the early stages?"

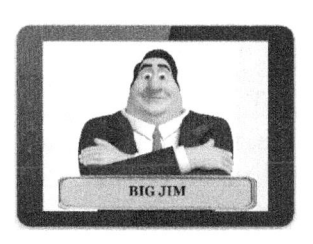

"Well! When CBT was first mentioned to me I felt a bit embarrassed. I wasn't really sure that I needed it. My wife and GP told me it would be a good idea, but I wasn't so keen. I went along for the appointment anyway. I didn't know what was going to happen. When I was actually in the appointment I realised I was glad I went. My therapist helped me understand what was making me feel the way I was. I felt so much better afterwards, and I seemed to be able to get a lot of things off my chest. "

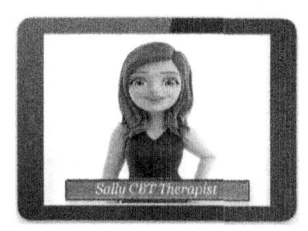

"Thank you Big Jim. Now the next person I would like to introduce to our readers to is Professor Harold Knutt. Professor Knutt is what people might call an **academic**. Academics spend a lot of time studying or researching specialist subjects at institutions like universities. Professor Knutt's specialist subject is the brain. In fact, he has spent so much time researching it at University he has been awarded five degrees, including two doctorates."

"Professor Knutt, thank you for joining us today. Many people like to know theories and scientific facts that explain why they feel the way they do! As we go on it will be very interesting to hear about any research you have come across that gives us further information about the things we are talking about."

"So Professor Knutt what might our readers need to know if they decide to do CBT on their own if they have CBT with a therapist?

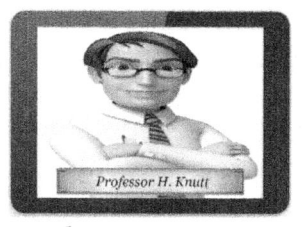

"OK, Sally our readers can find lots of useful information about CBT in books, not unlike like this one. Our readers can also go online and watch videos on YouTube, some of which I will direct them to in this book. Sometimes, however, working through books and video's is not enough on its own, or it does not change things quickly enough. If this is the case, our readers may decide to meet with a **registered therapist**. Registered therapists are members of professional bodies. These are organisations that check out all their therapists to make sure that they have the required training to do their jobs properly, and to work safely with people. There are many different professional bodies and therapists usually display a certificate in a frame to let their clients know which ones they belong to. If our readers decide to meet with a registered therapist they might need to know that their therapist will be highly trained and professional. Each therapist will recognise that when their clients attend therapy for the first time it will be important for their clients to have a positive experience and to feel safe."

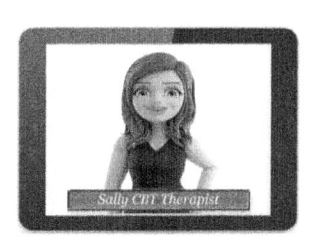

"What types of professionals offer CBT?"

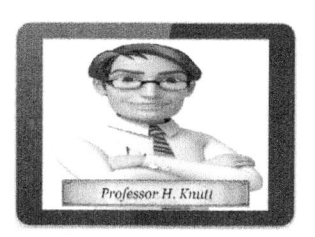

"Many professionals are now trained in CBT. Most Clinical Psychologists and Counselling Psychologists, in particular, are trained in it and tend to offer it. If our readers meet with a psychologist, they will be meeting somebody with extensive training, who is likely to have come across the types of problems that they may want to talk about many times before. Their training requires them to complete a degree in Psychology, a further advanced degree in psychology or to work as an Assistant Psychologist for at least a year, and they usually complete a Doctorate in the final 3 to 4 years of their training. From beginning to end their initial training can take between 6 and 9 years. For Consultant Psychologists their training period is at least 14 years. By the end of their training they have learned how to put people at ease and will fully understand the scientific principles behind the therapy that they offer."

Chapter 2

What you will learn about the brain in the early stages of therapy

"Many people go to therapy with specific problems that are concerning them. Some people may feel *anxious, stressed, depressed, have problems in their relationships* or find it difficult to cope with life in general."

"Sharing some information about how the brain works before they start therapy may benefit our readers. Let's start with you Big Jim. What did you find out about the brain?"

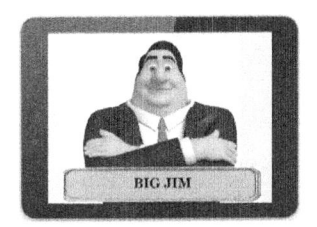

"There are three parts to the brain that you will find out about when you do CBT. The clever part is based at the top of the brain."

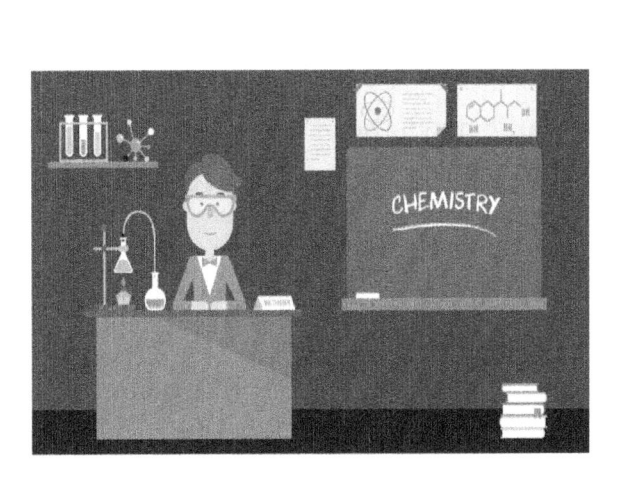

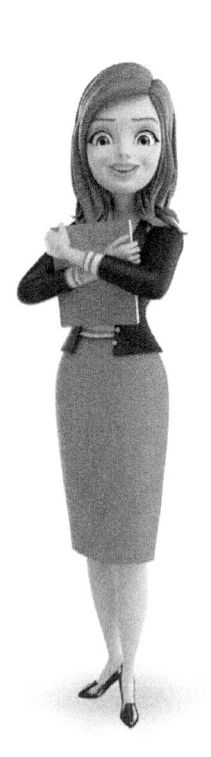

"The clever part is better at doing difficult things like crosswords, mathematics and solving problems."

"At the bottom of the brain is the animal part."

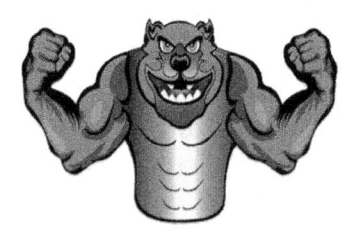

"The animal part is very loyal, a bit like my dog, but is also pretty gullible and believes everything that you tell it. It is in charge of feelings so we need to be careful with it. There is another little part in between the clever part and the animal part. It sorts out problems between the two of them. This part is the "minder.""

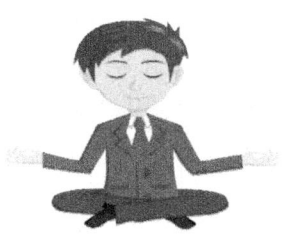

"The minder helps the brainy part sort out the animal when it gets a bit upset or angry. The minder is very good at calming down the animal part and can manage it, if it gets agitated."

THE ANIMAL

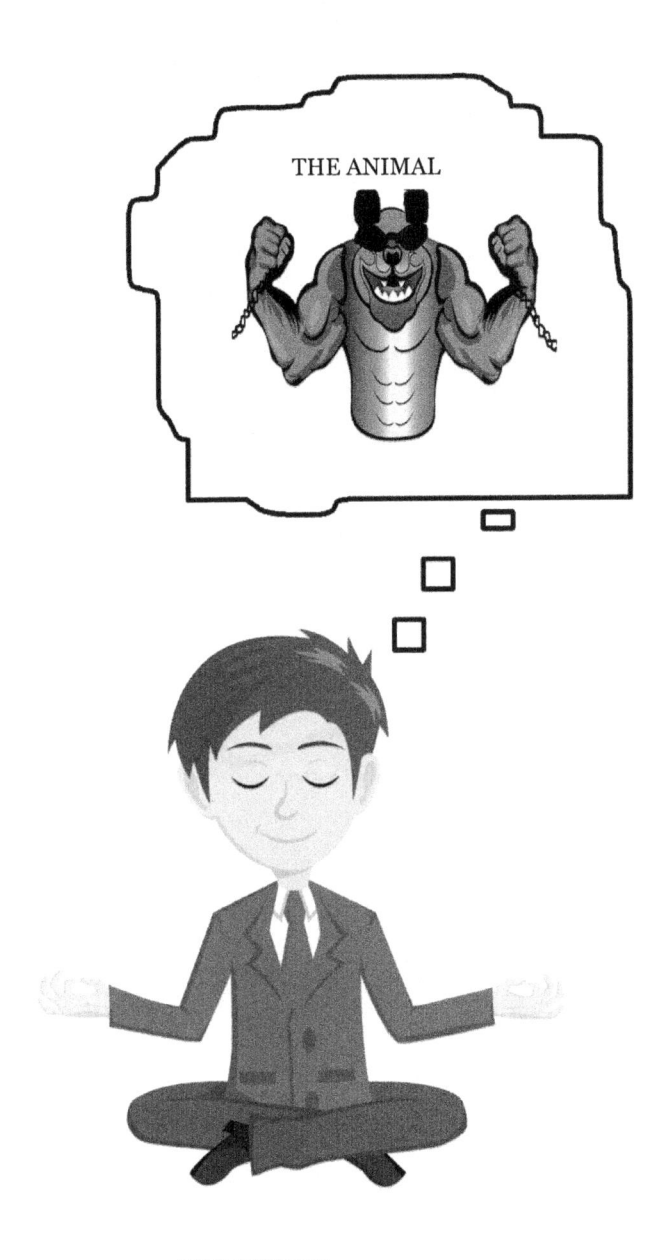

THE MINDER

"Overall the brain is structured a bit like the picture I have drawn below."

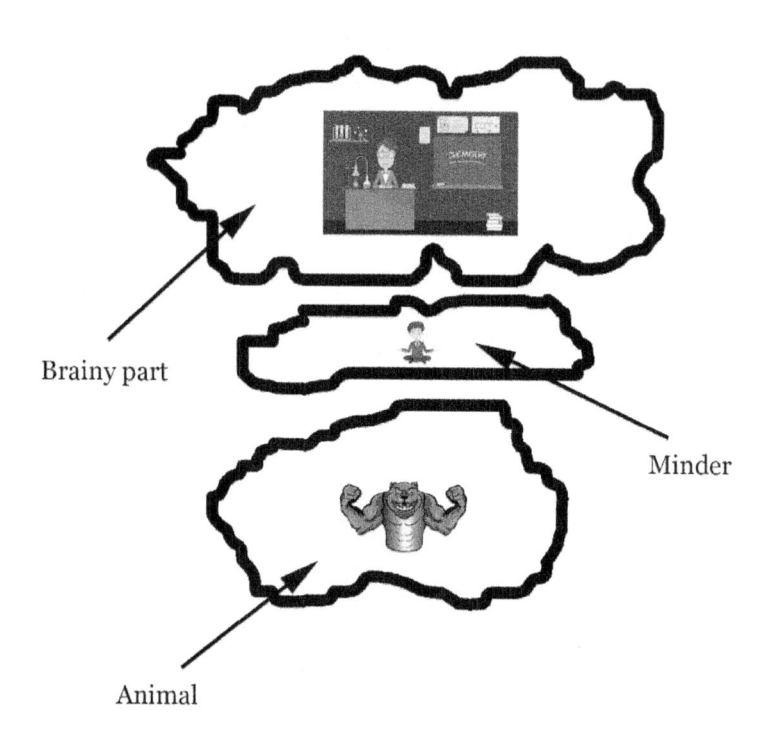

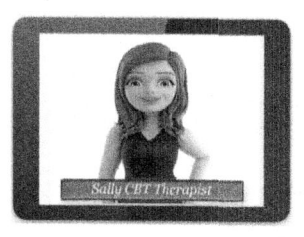

Brainy part

Minder

Animal

"Professor Knutt. Do you have anything to add about what people might find out about the brain?"

Sally CBT Therapist

"Have a look at my diagram overleaf. If you look at the brain from the top down everything that you can see on the surface is called the **neo-cortex**. The neo-cortex is a part of the brain that we use to think, plan and solve complex problems. You will need to use this part of the brain quite a bit when

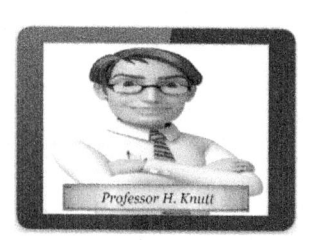

Professor H. Knutt

you do CBT. The lower areas of the brain that reside underneath the neo-cortex are known as **sub-cortical regions**. The sub-cortical regions could be described as the primitive or animal brain, as we share similar brain structures with mammals. This part of the brain is mainly interested in survival. The sub-cortical region is where our emotional reactions start."

The sub-cortical regions contain an area of the brain known as the limbic system. The limbic system and the area beneath it are where emotions are generated. The Amygdala in particular, which is located on both sides of the brain, triggers emotions such as anxiety. I will talk more about these parts of the brain later on."

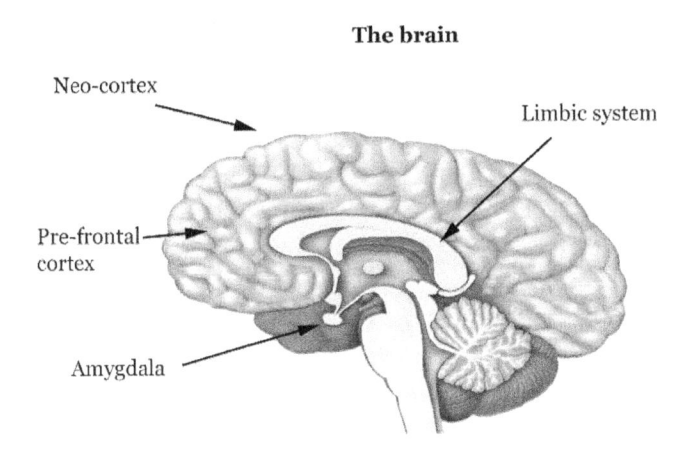

The brain

"I think the part of the brain that Big Jim calls 'the minder' is technically known as the **pre-frontal cortex**. The pre-frontal cortex is an extremely important part of the brain in terms of human evolution. It acts as a messenger between the neo-cortex and the primitive brain regions that lie beneath it."

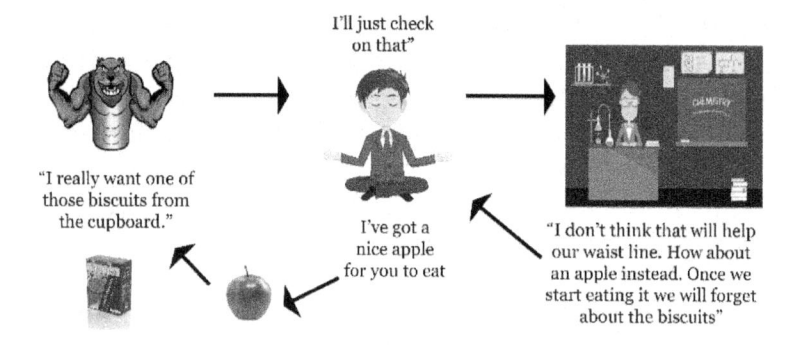

"I really want one of those biscuits from the cupboard."

"I'll just check on that"

"I've got a nice apple for you to eat"

"I don't think that will help our waist line. How about an apple instead. Once we start eating it we will forget about the biscuits"

"The pre-frontal cortex sits on top of the limbic system and acts as a communication system between the neo-cortex and the sub-cortical region. It has many important jobs. It quietens down noise in the mind and it can call off emotional reactions created by sub-cortical regions. We also use this part of our brain to think about our thinking. I've just added a few notes to Big Jim's picture and put it on the next page."

Brainy part
Neo-cortex

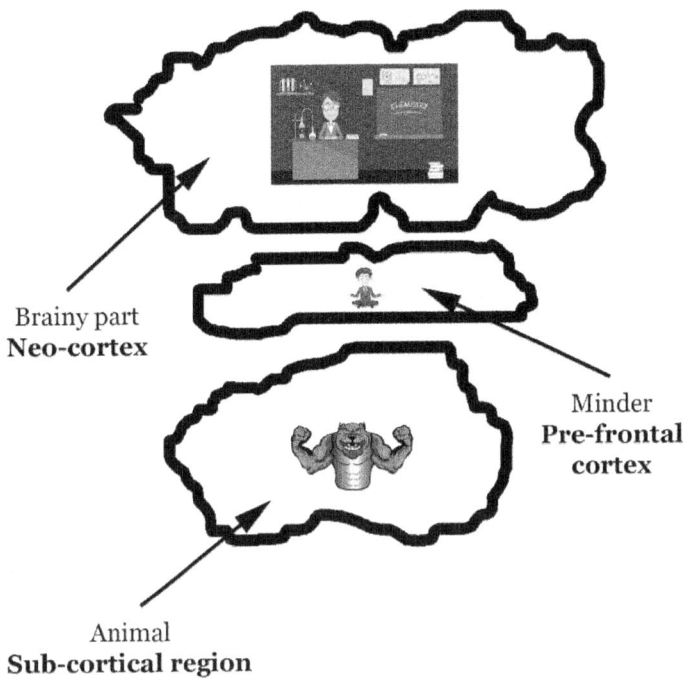

Minder
Pre-frontal cortex

Animal
Sub-cortical region

Chapter 3

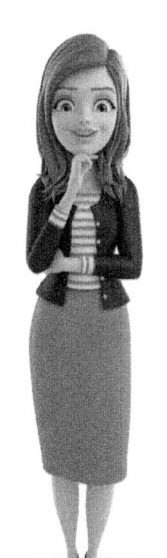

Thoughts affect the way that we feel

"Most people who attend CBT find out that the way that they think affects the way that they feel. Therapists help their clients to identify their thoughts and what happens in their body when they have these thoughts. So Jemma how is it that thoughts affect the way that you feel?"

"Basically the animal part listens in to all of your thoughts. It likes to be ready and prepared for whatever it thinks you might want to do next. It's a bit like my neighbour's dog when he goes for a walk. He pulls at his lead chocking himself. He doesn't know where he's going, but he always wants to be first."

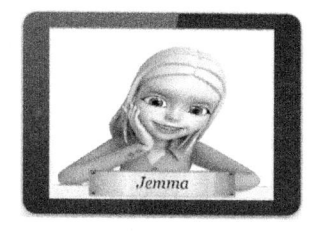

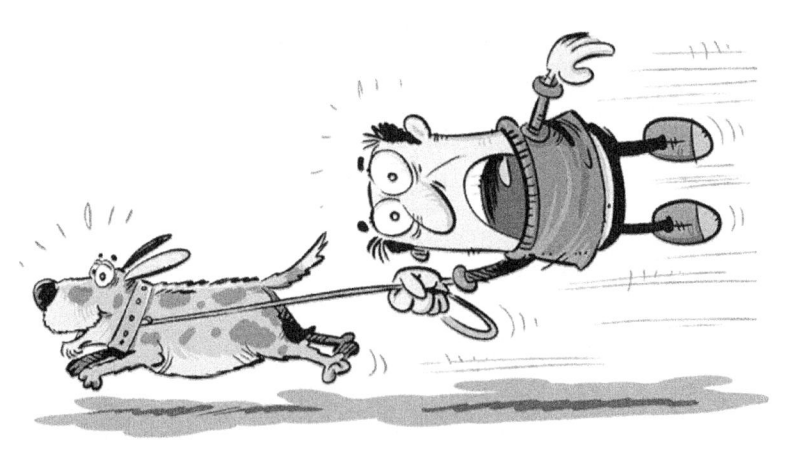

"Hey wait! I said it's getting dark...Not park!"

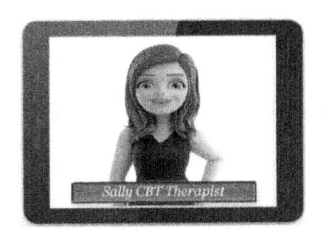

"So can you tell us anything about the science behind this Professor Knutt?"

"The brain works **holistically.** By holistic I mean most parts work at the same time or in parallel and they are directly connected to other parts. Information travels through the brain in microseconds. As a result of this, the subcortical region of the brain where emotions spring from have access to every thought that occurs within the mind very quickly. Not all thoughts generate feelings. The main thoughts that generate feelings are those that are more directly linked to our survival as humans. Thoughts connected to our social conduct, our financial future, reproduction, physical security, friendships, family, food, and social status are more likely to generate emotions. Emotions are basic survival mechanisms that helped our ancestors survive and they are really why we are here today."

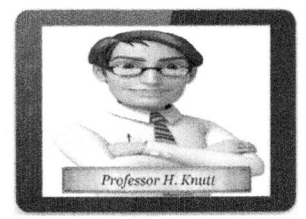

Chapter 4

What makes us have distressing feelings when we think we shouldn't have them?

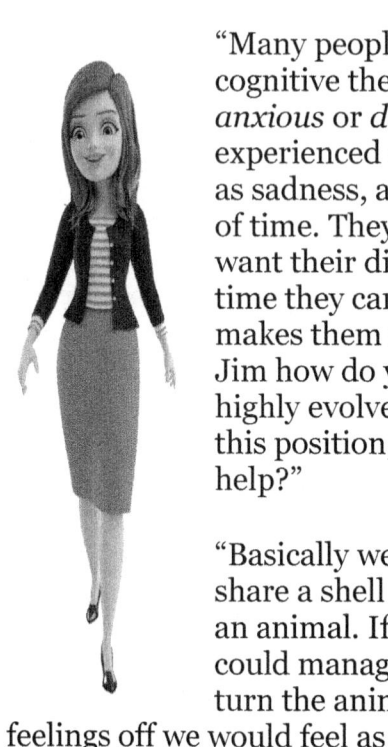

"Many people who choose to have cognitive therapy do so because they are *anxious* or *depressed*. They may have experienced distressing emotions such as sadness, anger or fear for long periods of time. They feel worn out by it and want their distress to stop. Much of the time they cannot understand what makes them feel the way that they do. So Jim how do you think we, as supposedly highly evolved humans, find ourselves in this position, and what can CBT do to help?"

"Basically we share a shell with an animal. If we could manage to turn the animal's feelings off we would feel as though we're not really alive. The animal is actually very sensitive and has a lot of feelings. If we over-control the animal's feelings it gets depressed. If we let the animal be in charge too much it gets anxious. So we have to manage the animal very carefully. The animal also likes to do the same things over and over again. This generally occurs because animals are driven by habits, even when the habits are not sensible."

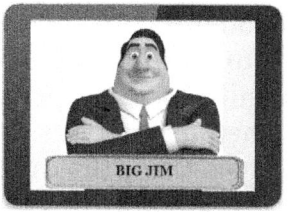

"My pet dog's the same. She likes to bite wheels on cars? It's one of her habits. If the wheels are moving she just can't help herself. CBT helps us to notice our unhelpful habits and to train the human animal into new habits. It's just such a shame that CBT doesn't work on dogs!"

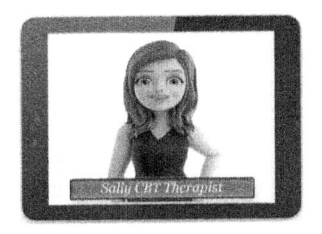

"Have you got anything scientific to add about this Professor Knutt?"

"I think Jim's right, as much of the time people can find themselves falling into repetitive loops or habitual behaviours with the way that they think, feel and behave. As a result of habitual behaviour, many people find themselves applying the same strategies over and over again to deal with their distressing emotions even when their strategies don't work. Traditional neuroscience suggests that the seat of habit formation can be found in the **basal ganglia**, a sub-cortical region of the brain. You can see where it is if you look at the picture below.

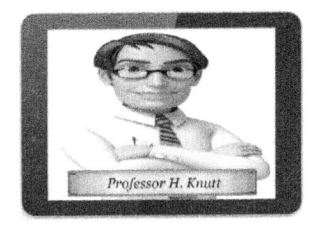

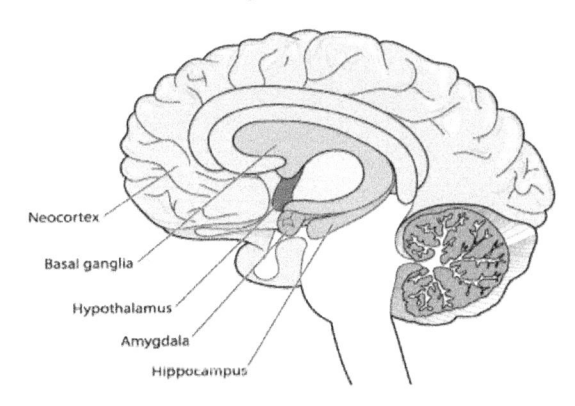

"The basal ganglia has been written about in great detail by my fellow professionals Carol Seger & Brian Spiering. I have put a reference for their 2011 paper in the back of this book, if you would like to read more about it. States of high emotional distress lead to primitive brain areas located in the sub-cortical region taking a central role. These brain areas are governed by habitual behaviour, which tends to be automatic, inflexible and rule-based. Habitual behaviour is generally thought to operate outside of our awareness and we revert to this quite strongly when we are under stress. CBT brings people's habitual behaviours to their awareness so that they can choose to do things differently. Breaking habitual cycles is not very easy because they are wired in, neurologically speaking to conserve energy. But! ... Once old cycles are broken, people can learn new positive habits. With repetition, these new positive habits can then also be stored in the basal ganglia and become automatic."

Chapter 5

What causes anxiety disorders?

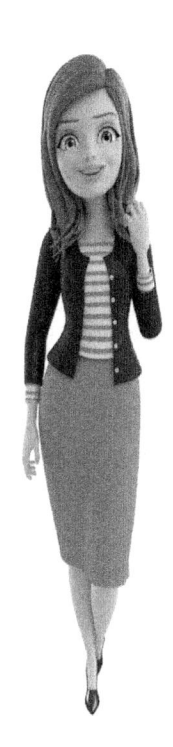

"Most people who attend CBT do so because they are experiencing anxiety. There are several different reasons why people can suffer with anxiety. They may have a diagnosis of *generalised anxiety disorder, panic disorder, health anxiety, obsessional compulsive disorder, or post-traumatic stress disorder* to name just a few. The list is very long and this book is not big enough to go into detail about any of these disorders individually. With this in mind, what's your general take on anxiety Big Jim?"

"Well, like I said before, the animal notices everything that is going on. It also sees everything and hears everything before the brainy part of the mind does. If we have too many frightening thoughts, it starts feeling threatened. If it gets really frightened or upset about something it has the ability to turn off the 'minder' off and take over."

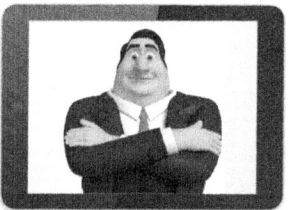

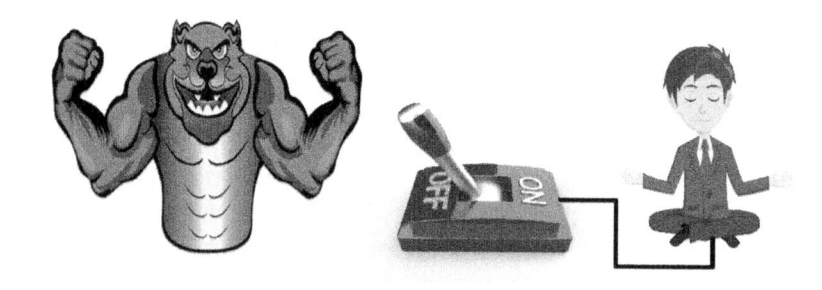

"I can't take it anymore. I'm dealing with this on my own!"

"Sometimes it tries to do the type of stuff the brainy part normally does, and hijacks the body. The problem is that although it's good at completing repetitive tasks, it isn't very good at anything that requires thinking too much. Sometimes this can cause more problems later."

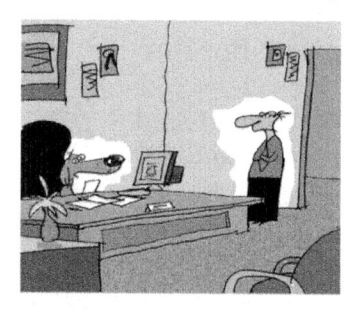

"Big Jim took the day off. I'm his dog, I'll be in charge of all his important decisions until he gets back. I'll just get the cheque book. How much did you say you wanted to borrow?"

"When the animal part feels frightened for too long, it gets more difficult to manage and the minder becomes worn down trying to keep it calm. After a while the minder struggles to look after it. When this happens too often the minder starts taking more and more time off sick and needs to take a break."

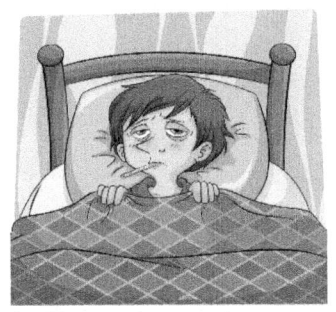

"I think I'd better take some time out to rest"

"With the minder out of action we start feeling more anxious about things that we weren't bothered about before. The minder isn't around enough to calm things down like usual."

"When the brainy part tries to do its job it can't think straight because its mind feels too foggy. The minders not there anymore to clear this part of the mind like it normally does."

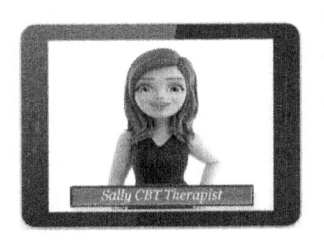

"Professor Knutt, will you be able to elaborate on anything that Big Jim has mentioned?"

"To explain how anxiety works, I'd better explain first about the passage of information through the brain?

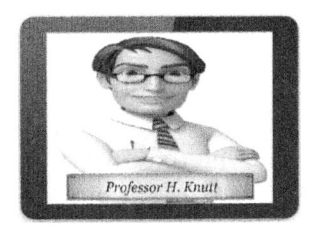

39

"Please do!"

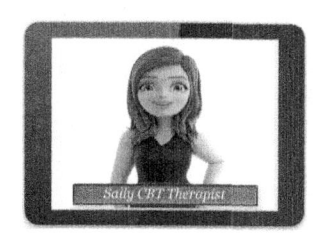

"All information carried by the senses passes through sub-cortical regions of the brain, before it reaches the neo-cortex."

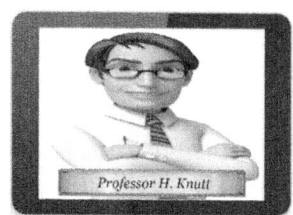

"When sub-cortical regions identify a cue that could relate to a potential threat in the environment, for example, someone shouting aggressively in the street, this can lead to sub-cortical regions of the brain triggering anxiety. If sub-cortical regions identify a cue relating to a threat that has occurred in the past, even if the threat is no longer valid in the current time mode, this can also lead to the sub-cortical regions triggering anxiety."

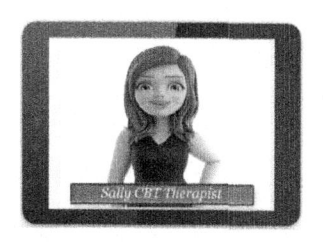

"I'm not sure I understand. How can something still be a threat, if the threat is no longer valid? That seems illogical!"

"Not if the threat is related to an old memory. Often the amygdala will trigger something called a **fight-flight** response to help the body achieve a state of readiness when it notices situations that have produced distress in the past. When a fight-flight response occurs the heart beats faster, blood is moved around the body very quickly, blood is moved away

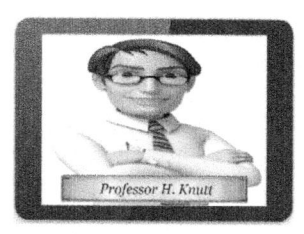

40

from areas focused on digestion into major muscle groups. This creates the experience that most people recognise as feeling anxious."

"In states of high anxiety primitive regions of the brain become more dominant as a result of the release of chemical messengers known as **catecholamines**."

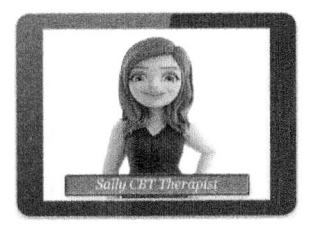

"Sorry, Professor Knutt, what are catecholamines?"

"All brain cells speak to each other using chemicals. Brain cells send out chemicals when they talk to each other, a bit like how we talk to each other using words. Catecholamines are a group of chemical messengers used by brain cells. The release of catecholamines improves the way that primitive brain regions function."

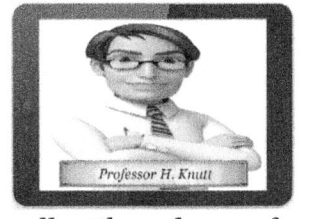

"Our assistant Debbie has a link below to a video for our readers to watch. This shows how the brain works."

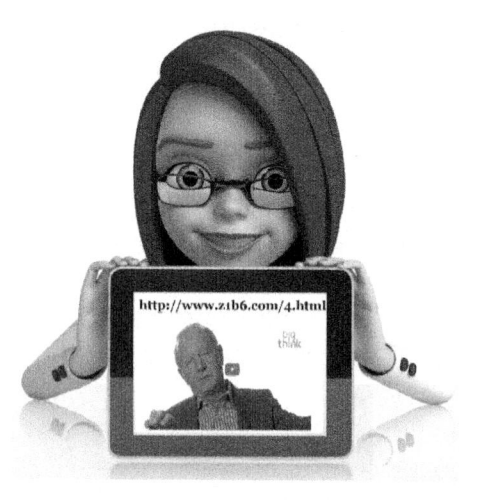

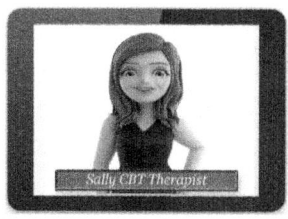

"It sounds like the release of catecholamines work a bit like a turbo boost or a power-up for the animal brain!"

"Yes, catecholamines certainly give the animal brain a boost. When primitive brain regions become more active, people become more aware of all of their senses. As a result of this, they may see, hear, feel, and smell things more strongly."

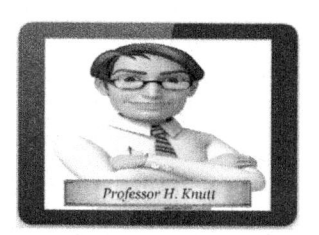

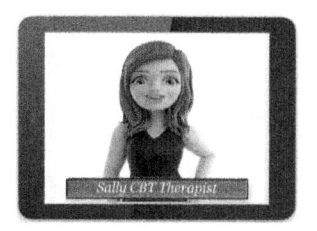

"Did you notice any of these things when you became anxious Jemma?"

"Yes, definitely. Everything seemed more sensitive. My skin felt hot and blotchy, my cheeks felt red-hot. My anxiety mainly occurred when I was in new social situations. When this happened I didn't feel myself. Things just seemed much more intense, mostly in my body."

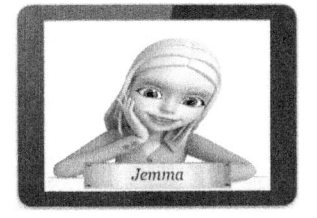

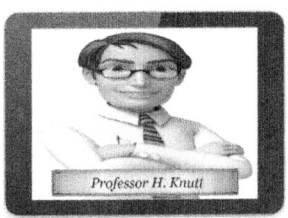

"What you are describing is exactly what the research suggests Jemma. In fact, in 2012 researchers Elizabeth Krusemark and Wen Li from the University of Wisconsin used functional magnetic resonance imagery (FMRI), which is a sophisticated brain scan, to find out how anxiety affected the senses, in particular smell. They found that when people became more anxious their senses became more sensitive."

"But, getting back to catecholamines. Catecholamines interfere with the normal operation of the pre-frontal cortex and stop it working properly. This interference is usually only temporary and when the threat dies down the pre-frontal cortex comes back on-line and starts to work normally as before."

"I guess that explains why people can't think straight when they feel anxious. When the pre-frontal cortex comes back on line they are able to think more rationally once more!"

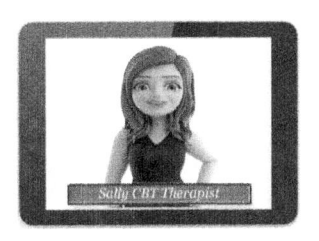

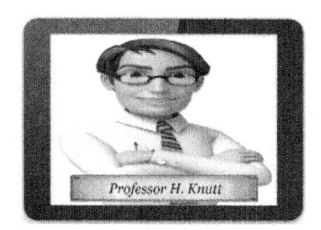

"Yes, you're right! The neo-cortex becomes less active due to the temporary disruption to the pre-frontal cortex! In order to think clearly you need to be able to hold ideas in mind, think about your thoughts at the same time, and have access to logical thoughts.

This is what the pre-frontal cortex enables us to do when it is working properly. When the pre-frontal cortex is overwhelmed by catecholamines it is hard to think clearly about anything. The same thing happens to my brain when I get anxious despite all my knowledge and education!"

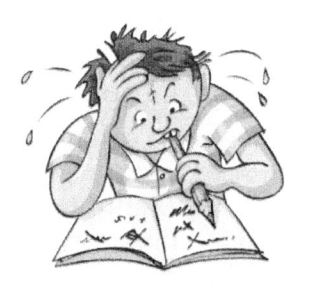

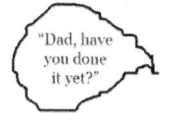

"I can't believe how difficult the homework for 11 year olds is these days."

"I have placed a picture of how this might work below"

5

The neo-cortex, or the rational part of the mind might know logically that there is nothing to feel anxious about, but can only observe. When the pre-frontal cortex becomes disabled it loses it's usual communication channel.

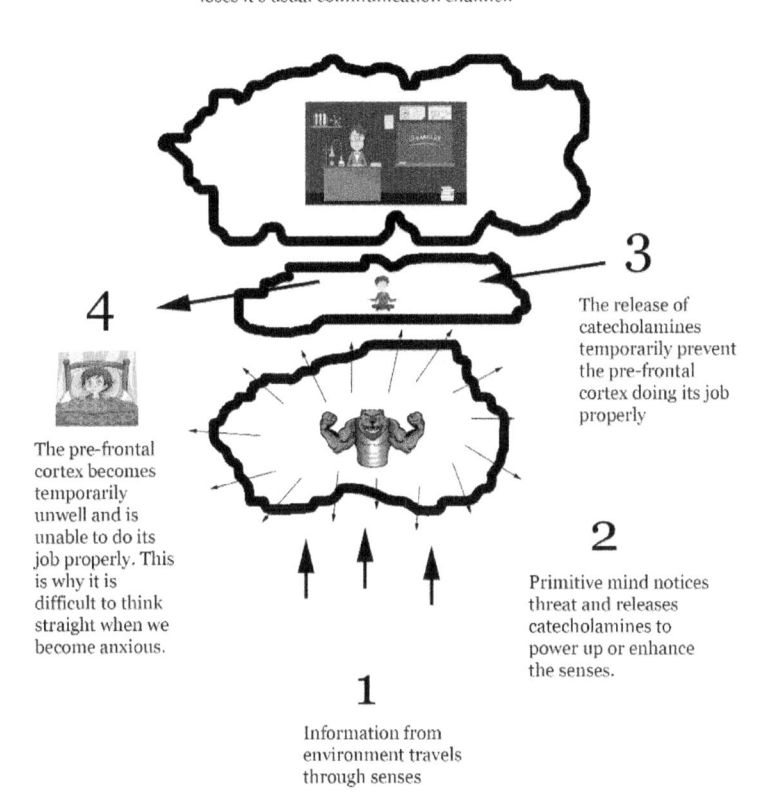

3

The release of catecholamines temporarily prevent the pre-frontal cortex doing its job properly

4

The pre-frontal cortex becomes temporarily unwell and is unable to do its job properly. This is why it is difficult to think straight when we become anxious.

2

Primitive mind notices threat and releases catecholamines to power up or enhance the senses.

1

Information from environment travels through senses

45

"When the pre-frontal cortex is working well it acts as a gate-keeper between the sub-cortical region and the neo-cortex."

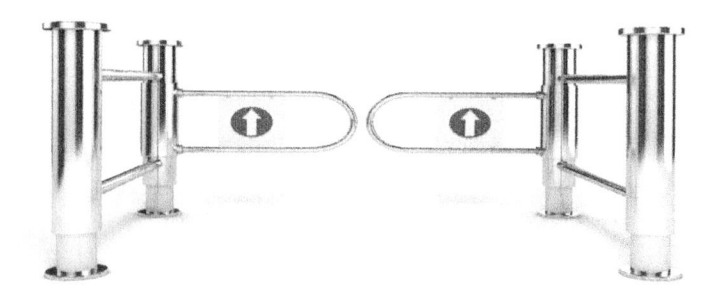

"When the pre-frontal cortex becomes disabled by heightened activation of the sub-cortical regions, the gateway becomes impenetrable."

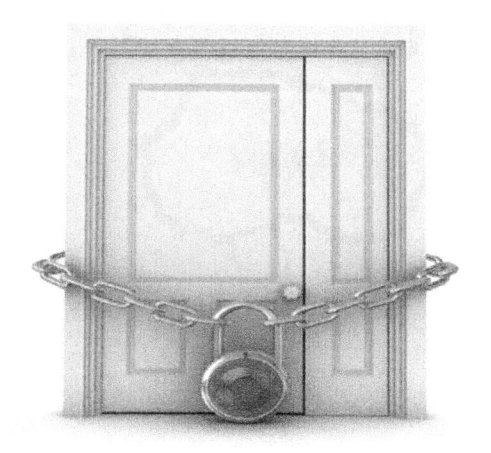

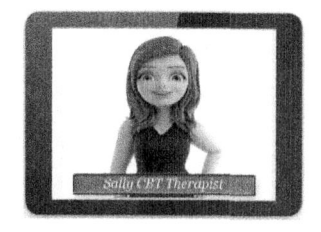

"We'll thank goodness it is only temporary!"

46

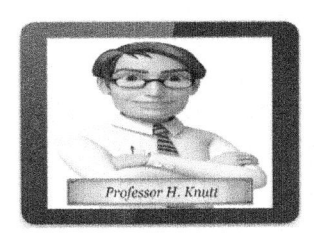

"Most of the time it is, but for some people the effect is more long lasting. I came across some research recently which suggests that when people experience stress for long periods of time, changes can occur in their brains. In 2015, Amy Armsten, Murray Raskind & their colleagues investigated several research studies looking into the impact of stress on the pre-frontal cortex. They found that a large number of studies clearly demonstrated that chronic stress led to a) reduced ability of the pre-frontal cortex to function as a result of catecholamine release and b) growth of the amygdala at a neurobiological level. Their investigation appeared to show that the longer an individual was exposed to chronic stress the less able they were to supress their natural fight-flight response and the more active their threat response became. This is why people with anxiety disorders can find it more difficult to manage their anxiety the longer they have it for."

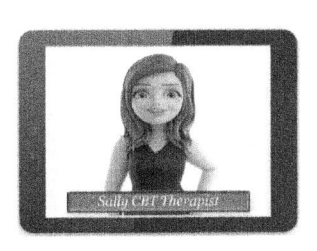

"What about people who worry Professor Knutt? How does this fit in with what you've told us?

"We know that when people feel anxious they worry more about things they would not normally worry about. The following ideas are my personal thoughts on this, so please do not quote me! I think people worry more because the pre-frontal cortex is less able to quieten down noise in the mind. Frightening thoughts are more likely to reach

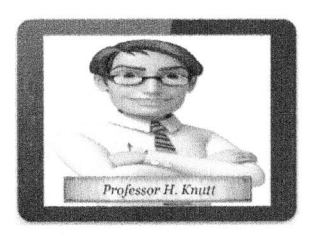

47

consciousness because the pre-frontal cortex is less able to screen them out. People worry more as they attempt to find solutions that they hope will help them cope with the feared situations or outcomes that are actually generated by their own worry process. Unfortunately, people's worry processes tend to keep them in an anxious position. Worry tends to generate even more frightening thoughts. This activates the sub-cortical regions threat responses even more and reduces the input of the neo-cortex. This effectively means that people are less able to think rationally when they spend too much time worrying."

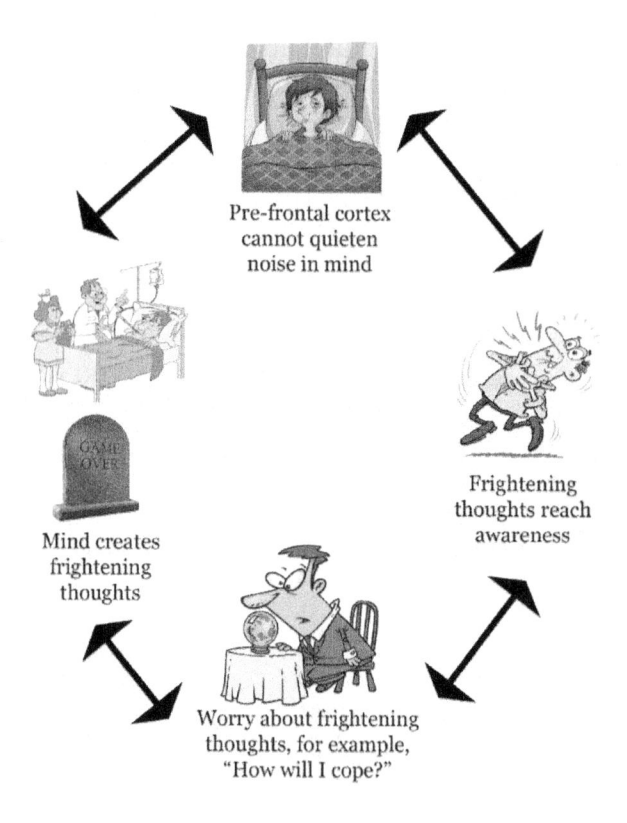

Pre-frontal cortex cannot quieten noise in mind

Frightening thoughts reach awareness

Worry about frightening thoughts, for example, "How will I cope?"

Mind creates frightening thoughts

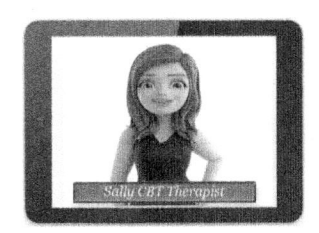

"OK...I think I might need to mull that over for a bit...It might take me a couple of days to make sense of that ... Oh...I think Kate is just coming online. I'd like to ask her what experience she's had working with people with anxiety."

"Hi Kate. I'm just having some live chat with some of our team. We're talking with Big Jim Smith, Jemma Jenkins, and Dr Harold Nut who you've met before I believe."

"Pleased to talk with you all."

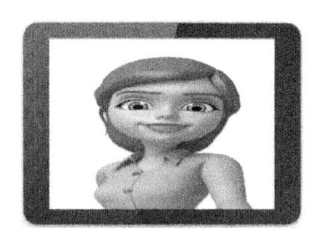

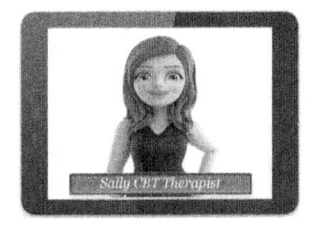

"We are just finishing off this chapter on anxiety and its impact on people and wondered if you could give us any insight into anxiety?"

"I can give you quite a general example of a situation that comes up come a lot."

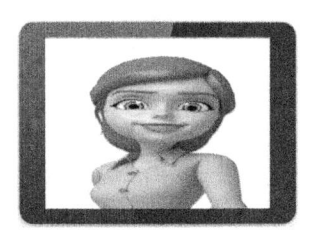

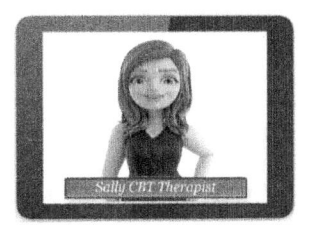

"Yes, please do!"

"Well, last week I had an assessment appointment with a surveyor. Let's call him David A. When he came into my therapy room, he looked flustered. I had noticed him earlier standing in our waiting area wringing his hands together, so I guessed he might be struggling with anxiety. Before I had even introduced myself he said "I'm so embarrassed to be here!" "I feel really silly!" "I may need to go" … "I hope you don't mind if I need to get up and walk out!"

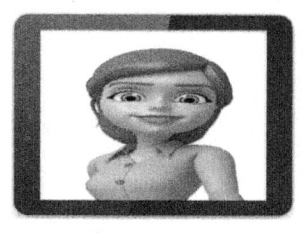

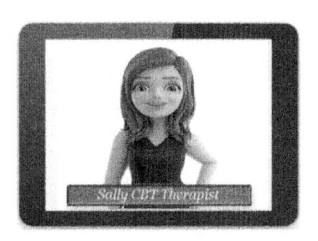

"So…Did he? I mean get up and walk out?

"Oh…No…He managed to stay with his anxiety…But he did get up out of his chair on a few occasions and walk around the room which was fine with me. Describing his symptoms and talking about them made him feel even more anxious. He told me his symptoms had come on suddenly while he was at work several months earlier. He appeared genuinely confused that his General Practitioner had told him that he had anxiety. He was sure that he was experiencing heart problems. Early on in our meeting he clutched his chest and began to breathe deeply, telling me "It's OK just give me a few minutes" as I asked him how his symptoms developed."

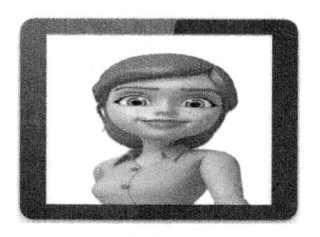

"As our meeting progressed I found out that one of David's main concerns was having a panic attack in front of others, and what others might think of him. He had been monitoring his body for potential signs of anxiety and it appeared that very minor changes in his body could escalate into panic symptoms very quickly."

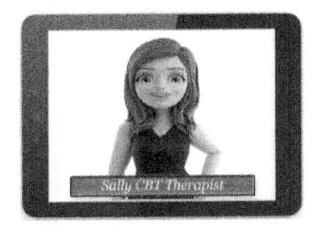

"That must have been very frightening for him!"

"Yes...It must have been. My initial thoughts were that sub-cortical regions of his brain were screening for changes in his body associated with anxiety and then firing off his fight-flight process in response to its own anxiety symptoms. He then started to become more vigilant to anything that might lead to him feeling anxious. This led to him monitoring his bodily reactions and he often took action quite quickly in an attempt to control his body's reactions and to clam himself."

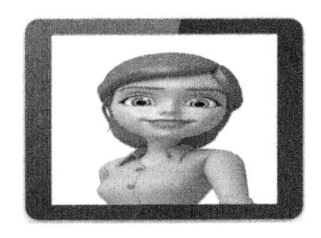

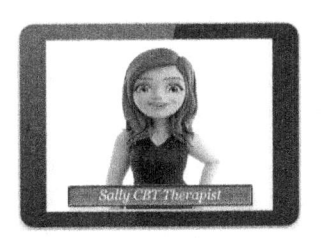

"It sounds as if he had a phobic response to symptoms produced by his own body." Is that what you would expect Professor Knutt?"

"Yes, that sounds extremely feasible. Memories of David's earlier anxiety responses could easily be stored as **unprocessed memories** in sub-cortical regions of his brain."

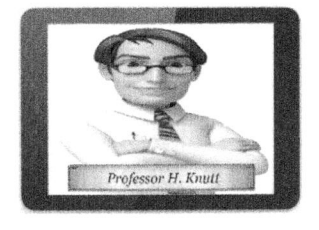

51

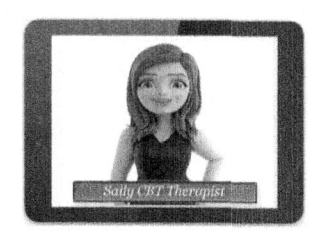

Sally CBT Therapist: "Sorry...I think we might need to explain what an unprocessed memory is for our readers as we have not mentioned what they are yet!"

Professor H. Knutt: "An unprocessed memory is an experience that the mind has not fully dealt with. At times a painful event can hurt so much, that people don't want to talk about it or even to think about it. They might try to block it out, because it is very painful to think about, or maybe there is simply no opportunity for them to talk about it. When this occurs the painful experience remains unprocessed and a memory of it is stored in primitive brain regions."

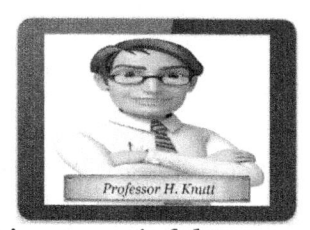

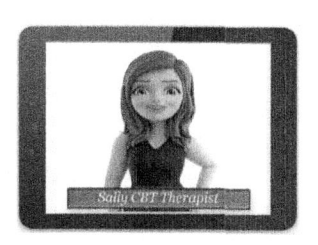

Sally CBT Therapist: "So what is the implication of the memory being unprocessed?"

Professor H. Knutt: "An unprocessed memory can sometimes create problems due to the place where it is stored. As I mentioned earlier, all sensory information, or what we see, hear, touch, smell and taste passes through primitive brain regions or sub-cortical brain regions before it gets to the analytical brain or the neo-cortex. In its journey through the sub-cortical mind, a part of the brain that is located there screens all sensory information for matches with past unprocessed memories or traumas. If

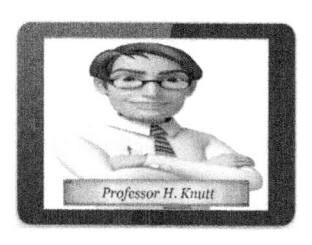

52

a match for an unprocessed memory is picked up, it triggers the body to produce intense emotions connected to the original event."

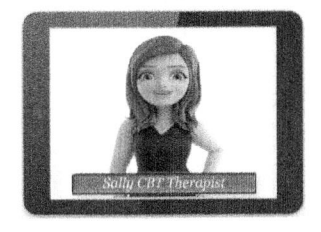

"Really, I didn't realise such a process existed!"

"Yes! It's a process that we share with all other mammals. I was listening to Professor Joseph LeDoux speak about it the other day. He has completed over thirty years of research on the mammalian brain. He told me all about it. He has quite a few videos on Youtube. They are worth a watch if you get a chance."

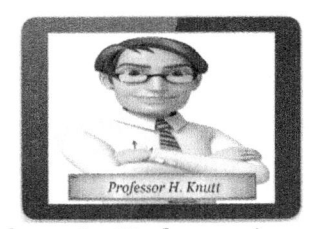

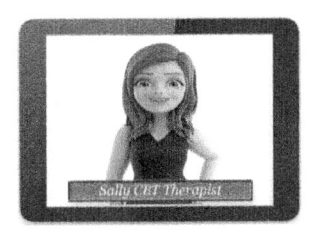

"So the sub-cortical region of the human brain or the primitive brain has its own memory system where painful memories from the past are stored and this triggers emotions in the here and now. That's quite amazing! Can you give our readers an example of how this works in practice?"

"Let's imagine that a five year old child is shouted at by a teacher in front of his or her classmates and feels humiliated. The child's primal memory system could hold this memory in an unprocessed form indefinitely. Anxiety may be activated many years later when the

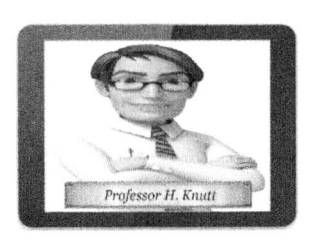

53

grown up child or adult is around authority figures that have similar attributes, for example, authority figures who shout a lot."

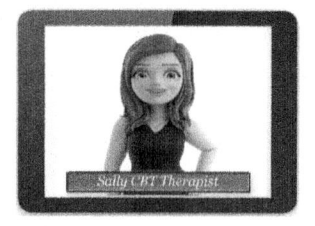

"So do people make this connection? For example, do they think to themselves - I'm feeling anxious around this this person because he reminds me of that teacher who shouted at me a lot when I was younger?"

"No...Most people don't make that connection. Most individuals are unaware that they are becoming distressed due to their past unprocessed memories. All they will notice is that they are becoming distressed."

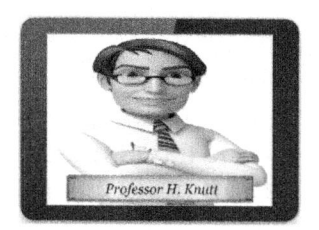

"So going back to Kate's example, If David A had a panic attack in the past, this may have left him holding onto an unprocessed memory it, as many people genuinely believe that they are going to die when they have a panic attack. Logically, he would fear being exposed to a similar situation again."

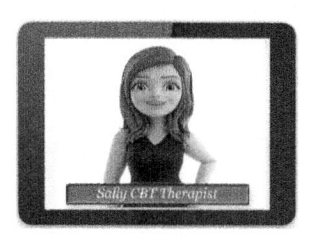

"So how did this affect him Kate?"

"David told me that he often monitored his body to see if his anxiety levels were increasing or decreasing. Following this, he used his anxiety level to determine whether he felt able to complete certain tasks such as being able to go to particular social events or to attend certain work events that he had in his diary."

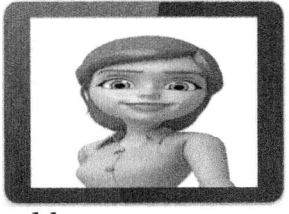

"David explained that as his anxiety symptoms progressed he took his anxiety monitoring to a higher level and he would try to monitor himself pre-emptively so that his anxiety didn't take him by surprise. He regularly began to monitor his heart rate by taking his pulse. He constantly assessed how his head felt, in particular how fuzzy his mind was. He had become highly tuned into his body changes viewing them as a potential threat. As time passed he had begun to make further associations about how he behaved and what might trigger body changes, such as rising from his seat too fast, walking rapidly, moving from a hot to a cold environment quickly etc. It was almost as if David felt that his panic was lurking in the background waiting to *attack* him at any moment and because of this he needed to be "On the lookout for it." David was extremely keen to know how to 'get rid' of his anxiety or to learn how to control it."

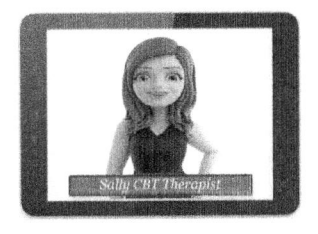

"What did you do to help him with that?"

"The main thing that I have helped him with so far is exploring an idea that attempting to get rid of his anxiety or trying to control it, in fact, only increases it further."

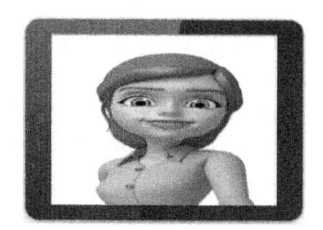

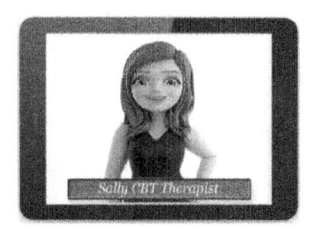

"That's fascinating. I'm not going to ask you any more about that now because as you know we'll be coming on to that topic a little later on in Chapter 15 and I don't want to spoil it for our readers."

Chapter 6

What causes depression?

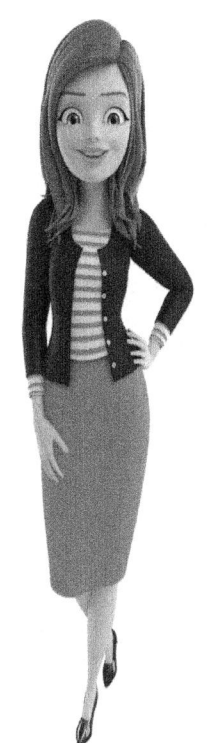

"Depression is a very serious mental health problem, and many people attend CBT sessions to work their way out of it. Like anxiety there are many different types of depression and there are multiple reasons why people can become depressed. In your experience Big Jim what makes people become depressed?"

"When I got depressed my therapist told me it was because my brain cells lost their voice."

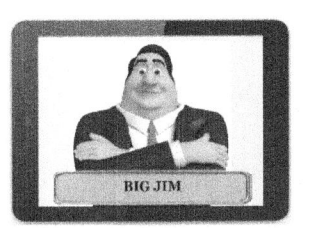

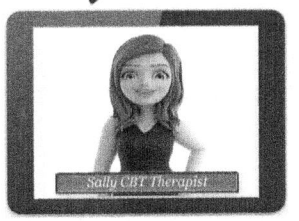

"Can you tell us a bit more about that Big Jim, it seems like an unusual way of describing how people become depressed?"

"OK Sally. I'll do my best! Basically the brain is full of cells. The cells all chat to each other using chemicals, a bit like we talk to each other using words. The way they speak is by squirting out these chemicals. When they've finished speaking they

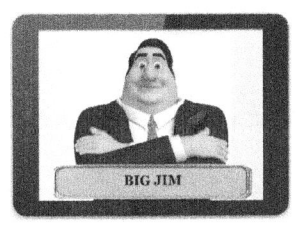

57

suck the chemicals back in to use them again later. People get depressed because the cells are talking too much to each about all kinds of negative rubbish and nonsense they don't really need to talk about. The cells then run out of chemicals and can't talk to each other properly any more. When the cells can't talk to each other, like they did before, the whole of the brain starts to slow down and we feel sad and lethargic. The doctor gave me some tablets to stop my cells sucking their chemicals back in. This meant that there were more chemicals floating around in my brain. It took some time for the tablets to work, but I did feel better after about 5 weeks."

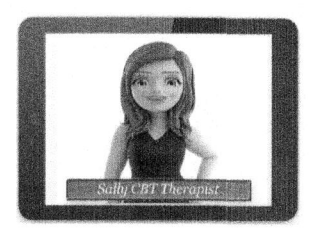

"And, Professor Knutt what is your take on why people get depressed."

"How long have you got? I have written whole books on why people get depressed."

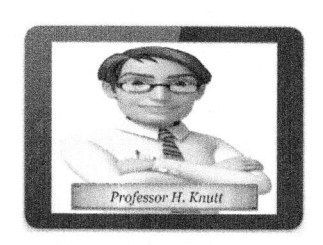

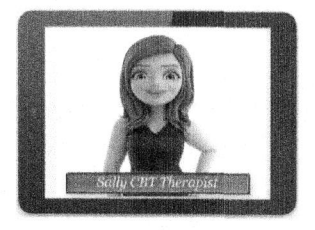

"Just give us an abbreviated version. We don't mind if you keep it short!"

58

"People who are clinically depressed are often physically affected by their symptoms for long periods of time, months or even years. Many individuals can experience a range of symptoms when they are depressed. Symptoms can include low mood, reduced or increased appetite, lack of interest in usual activities, poor concentration, increased or reduced sleep, reduced sexual activity, hopelessness, lack of energy, increased pain perception, thoughts of suicide, feelings of worthlessness, feelings of not being able to function, feeling slowed down, and increased irritation. People who experience depression can notice these feelings at different levels ranging from mild to severe. It is usually the severity and duration of the symptoms that determines whether a depressive episode is classified as mild, moderate or severe by mental health professionals. Many people with mild depression can function reasonably well in their day to day lives and the depression will often lift by itself without professional help. Severe depression on the other hand, rarely goes away by itself, is taken very seriously by mental health professionals and is viewed as an illness."

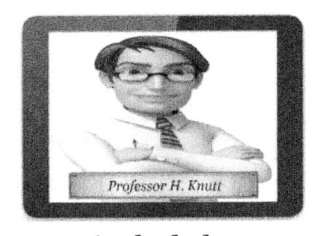

"People who experience depression will normally have the above symptoms for a period of at least two weeks. Bear in mind you do not need to have all of the above symptoms to be depressed. In fact, the majority of people who experience depression can do so without noticing a lack of energy or concentration, and can still achieve pleasure from things. This can often be very difficult even for mental health specialists to diagnose. Psychiatrists commonly refer to this as *non-melancholic depression*."

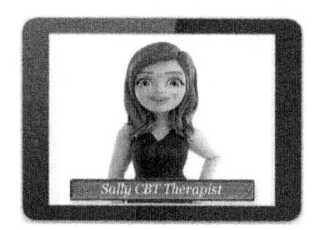

"Yes, I have come across it quite a lot in my clinical work. Many of these individuals don't actually realise that they are depressed. It is only when they come out of their depression by taking medication or by having therapy that they then really notice how depressed they were. So how many types of depression are there?"

"You probably know this already Sally, because you have borrowed my book written by the American Psychiatric Association on many occasions. For our readers benefit the book is called the Diagnostic and Statistical Manual of Mental Disorders or DSM-V for short."

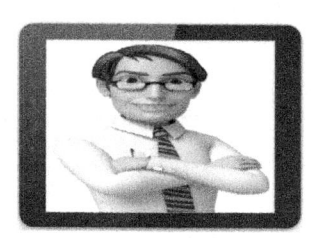

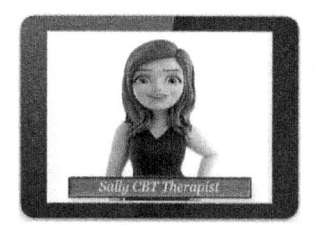

"Yes, I've leafed through it a few times. I've seen them for sale over the internet, I only borrow yours because I think I would need to get a mortgage to buy one! Can you tell our readers what it's for?"

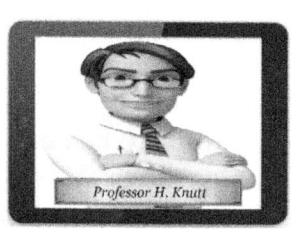

"The DSM-V is a way of grouping together symptoms into various subgroups and categorising them. Psychiatrists collect from all over the word to make decisions on the contents of this book and to determine what symptoms grouped together can be classified as a disorder. I am informed by my esteemed Psychiatrist colleagues that these occasions are often intense, heated affairs and that many suggested 'disorders' do not reach the final manuscript as there needs to be general agreement by Psychiatrists, many of whom don't particularly get on with each other. Thus far the DSM-V has over 40 different ways of classifying depression, if bi-polar disorder is included."

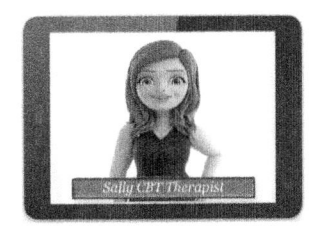

"So what are the main causes for it?"

"I've just competed a quick search for you on Google, Sally and if you look through the main medical websites you will notice that the medical writers find it very difficult to describe any single factor that causes depression. They are very good at describing the many different types of depression that we can suffer from and categorising it. The DSM-V is evidence of that. They are also very good at identifying the risk factors. Whether this is difficulties in childhood, head injury, genetic factors, problems in personality, medical illness, and hormonal changes to name just a few."

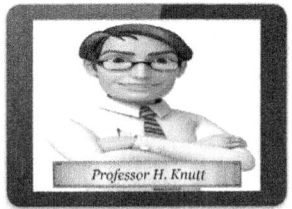

"In reality, however, there seems to be no simple answer that explains why depression occurs in one individual and not in another. It appears that depression is far too complex for that. Perhaps more realistically there are so many types of depression and so many different causal factors that thinking about depression as a single problem is highly misleading."

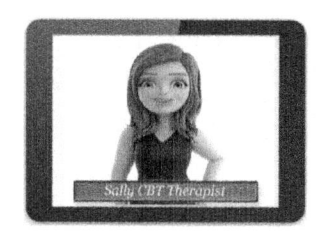

"So how do we need to be thinking about it?"

"I think the way we need to think about depression is as **self-perpetuating** problem. By self-perpetuating, I mean once an individual begins to experience symptoms of depression, the symptoms alone can fuel further depression. In this respect, once depression is active it has an ability to keep itself going for months, years or even decades."

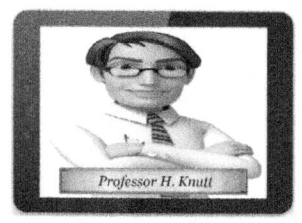

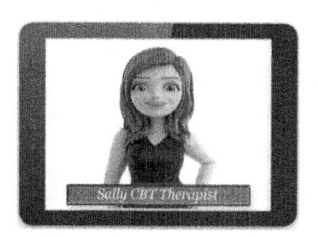

"Maybe you could tell us how it self-perpetuates?"

"Depression can have a significant harmful impact on the workings of the brain through a combination of neurological, biological, cognitive and behavioural factors. These factors essentially keep symptoms in place."

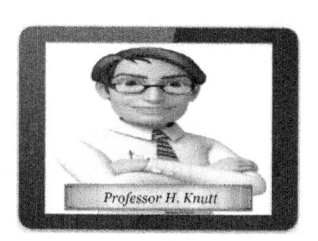

"People with depression can experience greater difficulties keeping healthy relationships with others. Attention and concentrating are affected which can lead to mistakes at work or at best slow down work speed. People who are depressed find it difficult to remain physically healthy. This can lead to self-neglect, which can have further negative health consequences down the line. They may also view information in an unbalanced way which can lead to rash or poor decision making that can have long-term negative implications."

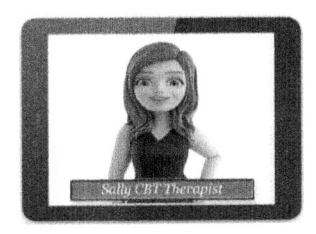

"Thinking about it that way I can imagine how somebody who was struggling with their relationships, making poor decisions, under-performing at work, and viewing the world in a negatively way might struggle to move out of a depressed position."

"I think we need to spend a bit more time on this area Professor Knutt as many people who have mental health difficulties and want CBT also experience depression. As you have said it can be devastating for them. So can you tell us some more of the science behind what you are saying?"

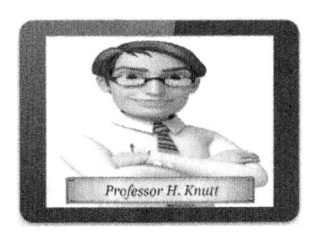

"Yes, I could talk all day about this. Let's start by going back in time to 2008. In 2008 the Archives of General Psychiatry, which is a prestigious international journal, published a very interesting study by Thomas Frodl and his colleagues. For three years Thomas Frodl's research team followed 38 individuals with major depression and compared them to matched non-depressed individuals. Over this time all the study's participants had their brains scanned on a regular basis using a process called high-resolution magnetic resonance imagery. Thomas Frodl and his colleagues found that individuals with depression had a decline in their brains grey matter, or in other words brain loss or brain atrophy, in specific areas. These areas included the anterior cingulate, an area devoted to conflict resolution, the hippocampus, a very small area of the brain used in memory processing and the pre-frontal cortex."

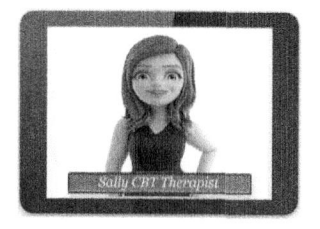

"Wow! I didn't realise depression could actually shrink parts of the brain. Didn't we talk about the pre-frontal cortex last time when we were discussing anxiety?"

"Yes, we did. As I mentioned last time the pre-frontal cortex dampens emotions, pushes down irrelevant or interfering stimuli, and helps us to think about our thinking. This has been known by psychologists for a long time. My old psychology lecturer Dr Brutkowski wrote about this 50 years ago in 1965. The pre-frontal cortex really is a very important area of the brain, as far as retaining psychological wellbeing is concerned."

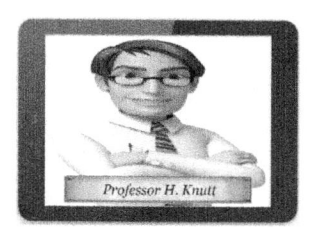

"Thomas Frodl's study that I talked about earlier highlights the important neurological implications of pre-frontal cortex atrophy on depression. In essence, a weakened pre-frontal cortex could easily explain why individuals with depression find it so difficult to detach from **rumination**, which is a process of churning negative thoughts over and over in the mind, even though many sufferers recognise that rumination maintains their symptoms."

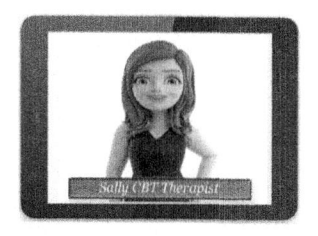

"Yes. I think most CBT therapists are aware that rumination maintains symptoms of depression. I work on **mindfulness exercises** with

64

my clients on a regular basis to help them detach from it. Mindfulness exercises involve staying in the present moment, bringing conscious awareness back to the present, and deliberately moving away from thoughts about the past or the future. Even when my clients have learned how to use mindfulness successfully it can still be very difficult for them to stop ruminating. However, I think this is too big an area to talk about in this little book. Professor Mark Williams had written a really good book on mindfulness called "Mindfulness: Finding peace in a frantic world" which I would like to recommend to our readers."

"Can we move on now and talk now about **serotonin** and 5HT? What do we need to know about it?"

"As a chemical messenger serotine plays a huge part in the body's overall physical and mental functioning. Although most people with depression may have heard that serotonin is located in the brain, less well known is the fact that most of our serotonin is actually found in our body's digestive system and blood platelets. Only 10 percent of our total serotonin is located in the brain. Brain serotonin allows brain cells to communicate effectively with one and other. Usually brain cells expel serotonin to talk to each other as Big Jim has already mentioned. They then suck the remnants back in to reuse later. You can see how this works by looking at my diagram on the next page. This is often referred to as serotine re-uptake."

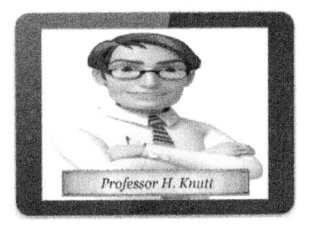

Professor H. Knutt

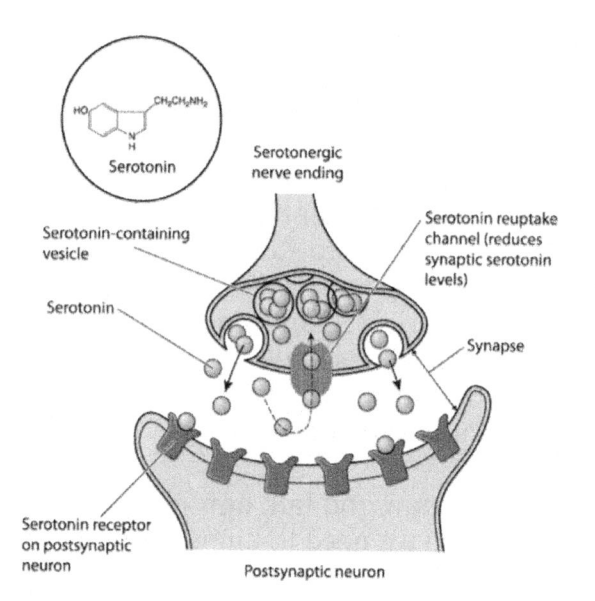

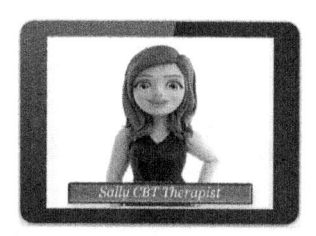

"Professor Knutt. While we are thinking about this, can you tell us how anti-depressants work, because many of our readers will be interested in this?"

"It's my pleasure Sally! Many anti-depressant medications are selective serotonin reuptake inhibitors, SSRI's for short. They work by blocking the serotonin reuptake process, more specifically by reducing the sensitivity of 5HT serotonin receptor sites or lessening their ability to suck back serotonin after they have released it. I have drawn another figure below which shows you how this works. When SSRI's work well they effectively leaves more serotonin floating about in the area between brain cells."

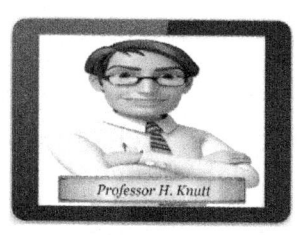

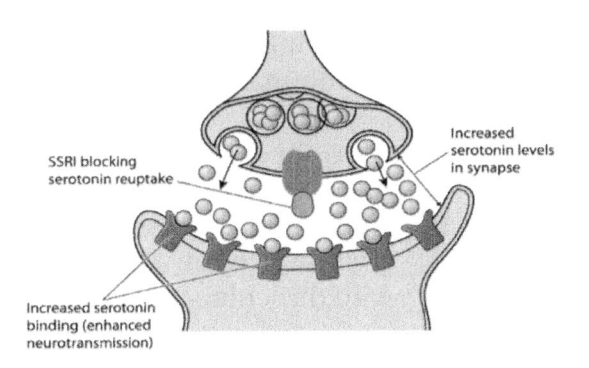

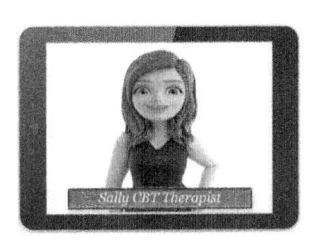

"So what actually happens when supplies of serotonin run low?"

"When supplies of serotonin run low our brain cells begin to lose their ability to communicate with each other adequately. As Big Jim mentioned, they 'lose their voice'. I have read some research completed by Dinan in 1994 which indicates that high cortisol levels, possibly brought about by stressful life events or indeed the stress of depression itself lowers serotonin levels and this is one factor that leads to depression. Other researchers suggest that individuals who are more vulnerable to stress, use more brain serotonin when dealing with difficulties and this creates a shortage in available brain serotonin and its **precursor**, tryptophan. By precursor, I mean the body uses tryptophan to make serotonin. Researchers suggest that this problem can be helped out somewhat by feeding stress vulnerable individuals a diet enriched with nutrients essential to the creation of tryptophan before they engage in stressful events, (Markus et al, 2002).

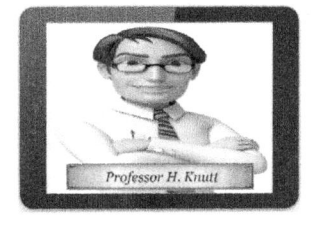

Apparently, Sea lion has the highest concentrates, but other foods such as, egg white, spinach, soy protein, seeds and sea weed also contain relatively high levels."

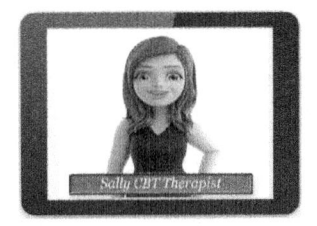

"I'm not sure people will realise that they are more vulnerable to stress and are using more brain serotonin when they are dealing with difficulties."

"Most people don't. A simple way of encouraging our readers to think about this could be ask them to think of their minds as like a household computer. Turning on their computer and then running every program on it all at once will generally slow down its processing speed. The same thing happens with the mind."

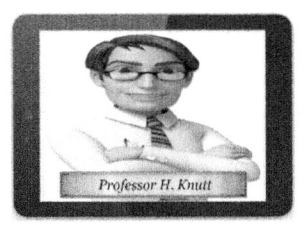

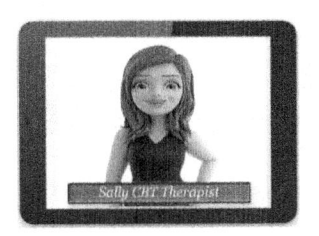

"So Professor Knutt, how do all the things that you've talked about combine to leave people feeling depressed?"

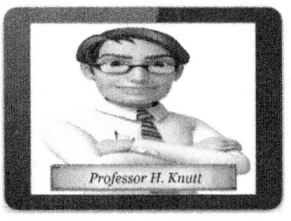

"As a result of many of the above mentioned neurological and neuro-chemical changes information processing is altered when we are depressed. Reduced serotonin levels lead to slowed mental functioning. Thinking becomes effortful, and problem-solving ability is not as good as was before. As well as this, reduced input of the neo-cortex can lead to loss of reasoned, balanced thinking which in turn creates an **interpretative bias** in the way that information is processed. An interpretative bias means that we filter information so that we only see want we allow ourselves to see, not what is really happening. I think we will be talking about this is much greater detail later on, so I won't talk about this now."

"With the pre-frontal cortex becoming less active, it has less ability to quieten down the chatter of the mind, which leads to increased likelihood of rumination. This will mean that more valuable neuro-transmitters are used on a mental process that generally achieves no positive results. With reduced input of the pre-frontal cortex this also means that there is less ability to be self-reflective, and attention, concentration and memory will be negatively affected."

"If you consider the above, all working together, it is not surprising that so many of us can find ourselves stuck in a negative cycle of depression. I have placed a picture of this cycle on the next page. The basic neurochemical and biological features of depression, reduce our ability to function, making it more difficult to climb out of a depressed state."

Cycle of depression

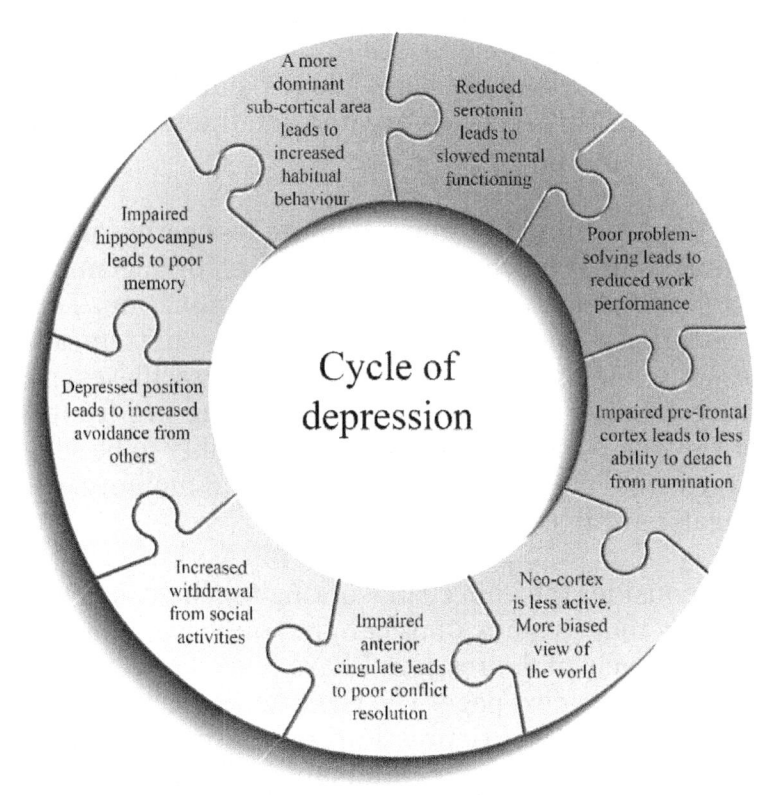

- A more dominant sub-cortical area leads to increased habitual behaviour
- Reduced serotonin leads to slowed mental functioning
- Poor problem-solving leads to reduced work performance
- Impaired pre-frontal cortex leads to less ability to detach from rumination
- Neo-cortex is less active. More biased view of the world
- Impaired anterior cingulate leads to poor conflict resolution
- Increased withdrawal from social activities
- Depressed position leads to increased avoidance from others
- Impaired hippopocampus leads to poor memory

Professor Knutt's cycle of depression.

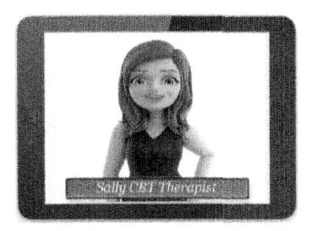

"I think I can see now why people can really get stuck when they are depressed. I guess with a more negative or skewed view of the world, people are more likely to want to avoid you. People who are depressed can lose friends or acquaintances, on top of their other problems. This is just likely to make their low mood worse."

Chapter 7

Avoidance and safety behaviours

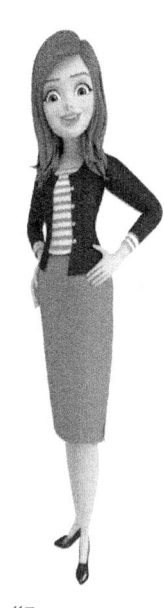

"The use of **avoidance and safety behaviours** are very common habits for people who experience psychological distress. Avoidance involves deliberately staying away from situations that might create emotional distress. People use safety behaviours to reduce their distress when they approach situations that they fear. Both avoidance and safety behaviours tend to keep people's problems in place and as time progresses continued use of them can lead to a gradual loss of confidence. Do you have any clinical examples that you can share with our readers Kate?"

"I once worked with Gregory, who was an energetic 26 year old, young father of two small children. He was an international I.T. expert and regularly travelled the world to give people advice on helping I.T. teams to work together more effectively. He was very highly thought of by his employers and he had recently been promoted to Vice President by his US based company. Along with his wife, and his General Practitioner I was one of the few people to whom he had talked about his difficulties."

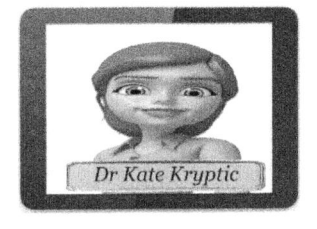

"Gregory's main focus in life was hiding any sense of vulnerability. Gregory told me that he felt panicky in many different types of situations, but did everything he could to not to show it. In his mind Gregory expected himself to appear confident, in control, able, sociable and intelligent at all times. In many respects Gregory described his life much like an acting performance that he needed to deliver perfectly day after day. When offering presentations he worried about his voice trembling and his heart rate rising. To cope with these problems Gregory took a beta-blocker, which is a drug prescribed for anxiety, before making presentations. To help him with concerns about his voice he recruited a voice expert to strengthen it. He had a developed several very clever rehearsed behaviours that he used if he noticed himself becoming anxious during a presentation. He had physical props in place that he could use, such as things he could hold onto. He had excuses pre-planned, which would give him an opportunity to leave the room for a few minutes. He had learnt how to do all of these things while coming across naturally."

"Around his friends Gregory painted a picture of himself as a confident person, again using a set of strategies that he had designed to avoid showing any type of vulnerability. Gregory didn't drink much alcohol when he went out socially due to his fear of saying or doing something stupid. He did not disclose any of his life difficulties even to his best friends. Gregory said that when he really thought about it the only person that he shared his fears with was his wife, and that even his best friend did not really know him."

"A particular problem for Gregory was that recently he had become much more avoidant about having meetings in person and had started offering **conference calls** instead. Conference calls are where people have meetings talking over the telephone rather than face to face. Nobody at his company had said anything about him doing this, although it was a particular source of concern for him, as being physically present with people was fundamental and expected of him in his work role."

"After meeting Gregory my initial opinion was that there was a lot of work to do with his anxiety as he had several avoidant behaviours and safety behaviours already in place. It seemed as though he was stuck in an acting role that he did not know how to get out of. He had become tired and exhausted as a result of his constant need to perform. I thought that he needed to become more aware of many of his many subtle avoidance strategies and safety behaviours before he could address the root cause of his problem which was his fear that deep down inside there was something wrong with him."

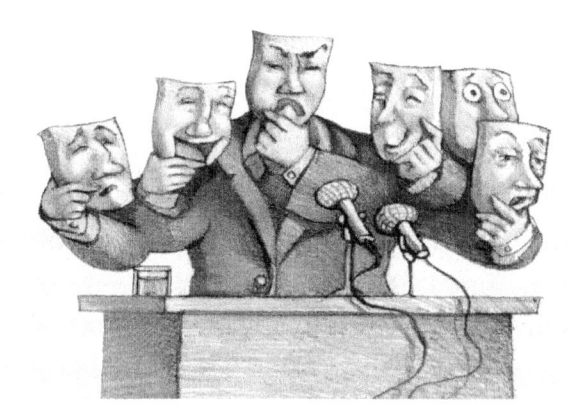

"I think that Gregory gives us a very good example of the types of avoidance and safety behaviours that many of us naturally develop to cope with life. Many people with mental health problems keep their problems a secret, and in fact, Gregory had hidden his symptoms so well over the years that it would have been a big surprise to others to discover just how anxious he was."

"Many individuals with mental health difficulties develop a range of imaginative strategies to control or avoid feeling distressed in all kinds of situations. Many people are skilled in finding ways to control or stop their feelings, and have become experts in developing strategies to avoid it or get rid of it. This behaviour is not surprising, not only due to our natural inclination to avoid high levels of distress, but also because it's normal to want to avoid potentially harmful outcomes."

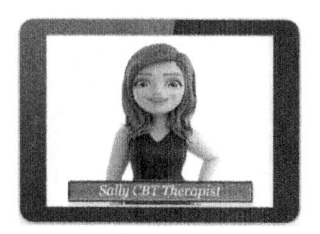

"So what impact do using these types of strategies have in the long-term Professor Knutt?"

"I think that there is a major problem with using avoidance and safety behaviours where emotional distress is concerned. The more we use safety behaviours, the more automatic safety behaviours and avoidance strategies become. It is natural for us to experience a sense of relief when we carry out a behaviour that removes pain or reduces worry. I have illustrated this in my diagram below. In psychological terms this process is referred to as **negative reinforcement**. Negative reinforcement occurs when we carry out certain behaviours to remove painful feelings. Over time, as processes are repeated and memory pathways are laid down we begin to engage in these behaviours automatically without thinking."

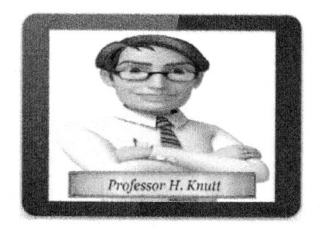

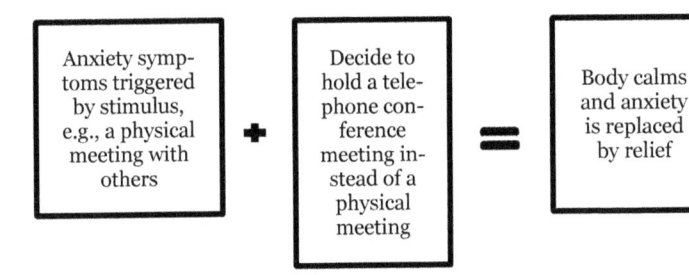

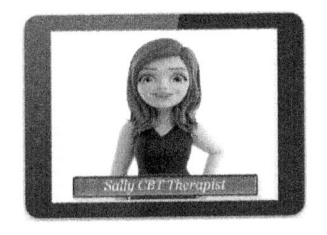

```
┌─────────────┐     ┌─────────────┐     ┌─────────────┐
│ Anxiety symp-│     │  Decide to  │     │             │
│toms triggered│     │ hold a tele-│     │ Body calms  │
│ by stimulus, │  +  │ phone con-  │  =  │ and anxiety │
│ e.g., a physical │   │  ference    │     │ is replaced │
│ meeting with │     │ meeting in- │     │  by relief  │
│   others    │     │  stead of a │     │             │
│             │     │  physical   │     │             │
│             │     │   meeting   │     │             │
└─────────────┘     └─────────────┘     └─────────────┘
```

Sally CBT Therapist: "What are your thoughts on Gregory Jemma?"

Jemma: "It probably felt to him that the more he used his strategies the less anxiety other people noticed in him. At first, he must have felt like he was dealing really well with his problem. As time went on, he must have started to feel more anxious than he did before. And, things must have got bad, as did end up seeing Kate eventually, didn't he?"

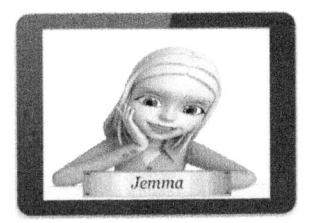

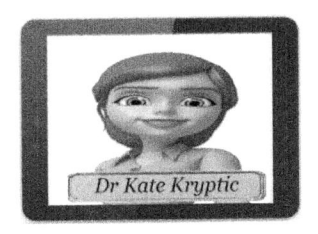

Dr Kate Kryptic: "You've hit the nail on the head there Jemma. I drew out a chart with him to describe what was happening. I have copied it onto the next page."

75

```
┌─────────────────────────────────────────────────┐
│              Trigger event                       │
│  e.g., anxiety symptoms at thought of a physical │
│             meeting with others                  │
└─────────────────────────────────────────────────┘
                       ↓
┌─────────────────────────────────────────────────┐
│ Anxiety response – Take action to reduce threat  │
│ by using safety behaviour e.g., change meeting   │
│ to telephone conference call                     │
└─────────────────────────────────────────────────┘
                       ↓
┌─────────────────────────────────────────────────┐
│        Temporary reduction in anxiety            │
└─────────────────────────────────────────────────┘
                       ↓
┌─────────────────────────────────────────────────┐
│ Changing social challenge is associated with     │
│ reduced distress                                 │
└─────────────────────────────────────────────────┘
                       ↓
┌─────────────────────────────────────────────────┐
│      Avoidance behaviour becomes reinforced      │
└─────────────────────────────────────────────────┘
                       ↓
┌─────────────────────────────────────────────────┐
│       Confidence in ability to cope reduces      │
└─────────────────────────────────────────────────┘
                       ↓
┌─────────────────────────────────────────────────┐
│ Increased threat monitoring due to reduced       │
│ confidence in ability to cope                    │
└─────────────────────────────────────────────────┘
                       ↓
┌─────────────────────────────────────────────────┐
│        Increased symptoms of anxiety             │
└─────────────────────────────────────────────────┘
```

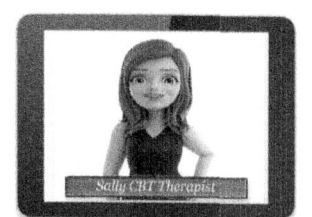

"Kate what kinds of safety behaviours are people naturally inclined to use when they are distressed?"

"I have drawn up a list of some of the more common safety behaviours and avoidance patterns that I have come across in my work. It's a very long list and it will go on for quite a few pages! If our readers have already completed their on-line assessment they can just skip to the problem that concerns them most."

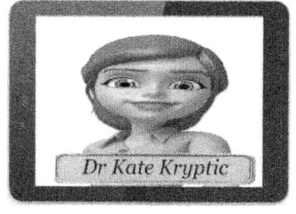

Debbie is showing a link address below for an online assessment for convenience.

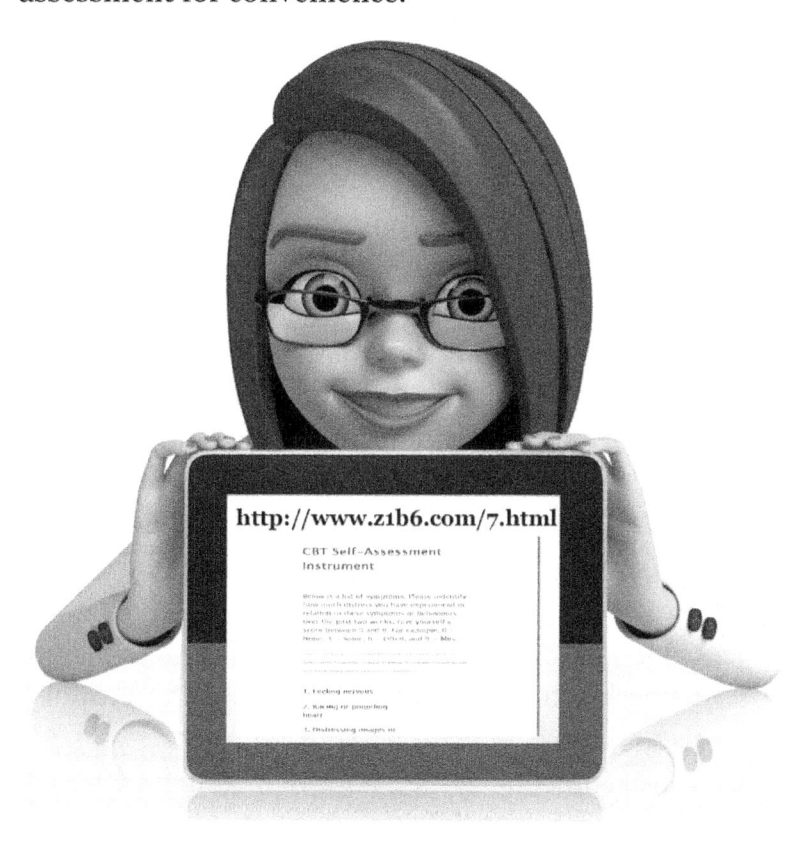

SAFETY BEHAVIOURS

Depression

- Say "Yes" to all requests
- Look for approval from others
- Compare self with others
- Withdraw emotionally
- Hide feelings
- Keep conversations short
- Turn down invitations
- Avoid confrontation
- Use drugs or alcohol to cope
- Ignore feelings
- Drop activities if not 100%
- Avoid conversations about emotions

Social anxiety

- Use diazepam or beta-blockers before social events e.g., business meetings.
- Carry a supply of diazepam just in case.
- Drink alcohol before going out to relax.
- Avoid situations where social anxiety has occurred in the past or where it may occur in the future.
- Go to the toilet before going out (related to fear of using lavatories and others overhearing lavatory use.)
- Have someone with you when going to social situations.
- Carry a bottle of water to help with a dry mouth.
- Sit close to an exit so as to escape unnoticed.

Social anxiety (continued)

- Hold onto or lean onto something supportive to hide shaking or trembling.
- Wear light clothing, fan self or stand near a window or a doorway to prevent over-heating. Alternatively wear more clothes to conceal sweating.
- Have tissue ready to wipe hands to conceal sweaty hands.
- Use heavy makeup to avoid others noticing blushing or cover face with hair.
- Drink out a bottle rather than a glass to avoid others noticing shaking hands.
- Have stories ready to put on an act of social competence and to have something interesting to say.
- Focus on self to assess social performance.
- Avoid conversations with people.
- Stand in a corner to keep a low profile.
- Keep conversations as short as possible to avoid revealing anything that could be self-incriminating.
- Focus on appearance.
- Try to control facial expressions.
- Avoid eye-contact with others.
- Mentally rehearse what is being said before it is said.
- Have excuses about a need to leave pre-planned and ready.

Anxiety & Panic attacks

- Use diazepam, a drug that alters neurotransmitter functioning to produce a calming effect, or beta-blockers before certain situations, e.g., using public transport, business meetings etc.
- Carry a supply of diazepam just in case.
- Do not move too fast due to fear of heart rate increase.
- Drink alcohol before going out to relax.
- Avoid situations where a panic attack has occurred in the past or where one may occur in the future.
- Do not eat before going out if related to a fear of vomiting.
- Go to the toilet before going out if related to fear of losing control of bowels.
- Have someone with you when in potential situations where panic could occur.
- Carry a brown paper bag to breath in and out of.
- Carry a bottle of water in case of dry mouth.
- Carry a plastic bag if related to fear of vomiting.
- Sit in places near to an exit in public places.
- Hold onto or lean onto something supportive.
- Hold breath, keep an eye on emotions.
- Fan self to stop self over-heating.
- Distract self, for example watch television.

Health anxiety

- Monitor any unusual symptoms in body.
- Seek reassurance.
- Make an appointment with Doctor or alternatively avoid doctors completely.
- Go onto the internet to complete research.
- Complete on-line assessments to self-diagnose.
- Scan body.
- Complete exercises to check if body is working OK.
- Worry about ability to cope with various physical disorders.
- Request medical tests from doctor or alternatively avoid medical tests totally.
- Request medical checks to rule out disorders
- Control diet.

Obsessional compulsive disorder

- Avoid situations or people that may trigger obsessional thoughts.
- Re-trace steps.
- Go back and check on things that you are unsure of.
- Complete ritualistic behaviour, such as touching wood to stop things from happening.
- Complete mental calculations, for example, the times tables to distract self from emotions.
- Push away intrusive thoughts.
- Complete activities a certain number of times.
- Perform activities in a particular order.
- Wear particular jewellery or make-up
- Carry certain items
- Check and re-check to make sure that you have not left anything behind.
- Look for reassurance from others

Obsessional compulsive disorder (continued)

- Stay with safe people
- Clean things to avoid contamination
- Hold onto items or hoard items

Phobic anxiety and post trauma symptoms

- Avoid certain objects or places. This may be related to something frightening that happened in the past.
- Avoid certain forms of transport.
- Take specific alternative safer routes when travelling.
- Avoid certain smells, sensations, tastes, physical feelings that produce anxiety.
- Ask for reassurance or ask others to check things for you.
- Go to places with safe people
- Avoid watching television programs about certain subjects.
- Try to be in control of others when you feel in an unsafe situation. For example, giving advice to others on how to drive, what to be careful of and such like.

Chapter 8

Self-observation

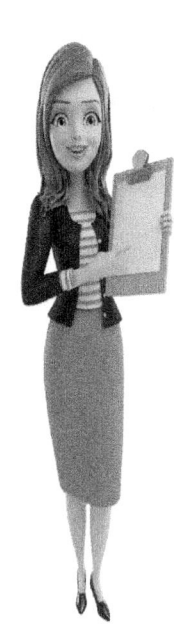

"Most people who have CBT will be encouraged by their therapist to observe themselves. The first thing they will be invited to notice is that they have thoughts and feelings. The second thing they are likely to become aware of is that they have a range of thoughts, feelings and behaviours in different circumstances. Once people become aware of this they will be encouraged by their therapist to monitor how they react in different circumstances. One way that people can observe themselves is by writing things down."

"What was your process of self-observation like Big Jim and what would you recommend to our readers?"

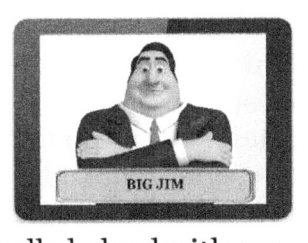

"My therapist struggled with helping me to write stuff down. The approach didn't really appeal to me. I thought that it might work much better for others. Eventually she convinced me to fill in sheets and I found that it actually helped with my mood. I noticed I could stand back from myself more. I started to realise I had many more feelings than I thought. I saw that a lot of the things I was doing in my personal life I didn't actually enjoy. I started to see that there were things missing from my life. I didn't notice this before I had therapy. Once I realised there was an animal part to the mind, I could see much more when it was around and how it affected the way that I thought. I noticed that the clever part of the mind and the animal didn't always agree. I started listening to both parts and then making decisions about my life after thinking about things in a more balanced way. The important thing that I would advise people to do is to start noticing the unhelpful thoughts and behaviours that they engage in much more."

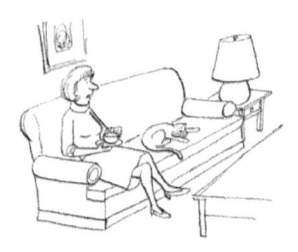

"The therapist says I've really made progress now that I've stopped talking to the cat."

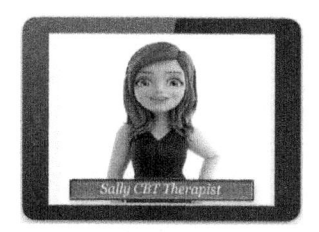

"So what difference do you think that noticing made Big Jim?"

— Sally CBT Therapist

"This is probably going to sound a bit obvious now, but I realised that for every thought, feeling or behaviour I had, I had a choice about how to react or respond. Before this, I was just living a bit like a puppet, acting automatically."

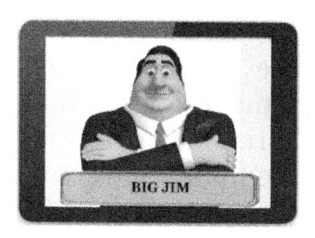

— BIG JIM

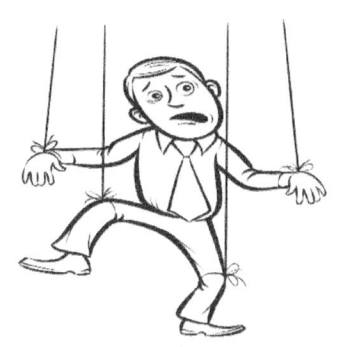

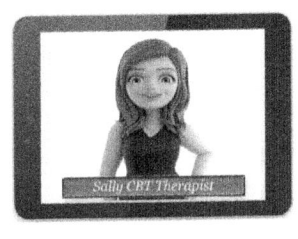

"Professor Knutt. Do you have any observations here?"

"Yes. I certainly do. Just as a professional running coach may recommend leg strengthening exercise to athletes to enable them to run faster, I am recommending to our readers that they focus on observation to improve the way that they feel. Observation exercises the pre-frontal cortex, and a stronger pre-frontal cortex is associated with improved **mood regulation**. Mood regulation is basically an ability to have some control over feelings. By beginning to observe their mood, becoming more mindful of how they feel, noticing or writing down their thoughts, and reflecting on what they notice our readers will be specifically working their pre-frontal cortex much more and thereby improving its ability to function."

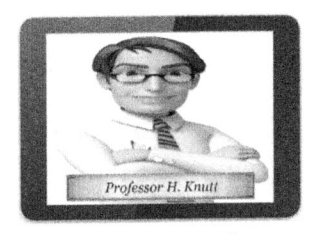

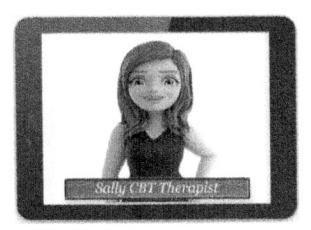

"This takes me back to what we were talking about earlier. Do you think observation can help people whose pre-frontal cortex has shrunk as a result of being anxious or depressed for a prolonged time?"

"Yes, I think so. The brain is well known by **neurologists**, who are medical experts in the brain, to have high levels of **plasticity**. Plasticity means that the brain has the ability to repair itself and grow in size the more that it is used. Neuropsychologist, Professor Eleanor Maguire from Ireland has published over 100 research articles and chapters on the neuropsychology of the brain. The majority of her research has focussed on memory, the hippocampus and the sub-cortical brain regions surrounding it. In perhaps, one her most famous papers in the 1990's, she and her colleagues reported results of their investigation into the brains of London taxi drivers. London taxi drivers were a very useful 'real life' experiment at the time, as there was a requirement that all taxi drivers complete a process known as the 'knowledge.' This required London taxi drivers to spend a large amount of time memorising the spatial layout of London Streets or exercising their hippocampi. If they did not pass the 'knowledge' test they could not become a London taxi driver. Eleanor Maguire used a process known as structural magnetic resonance imagery, a type of brain scan, to measure the hippocampal sizes of London Taxi Drivers. She found that London taxi drivers had significantly larger hippocampi than matched non-taxi drivers of a similar level of intelligence, and the more experience a taxi driver had, the larger their hippocampus was."

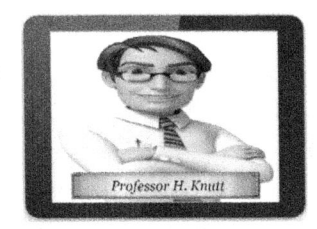

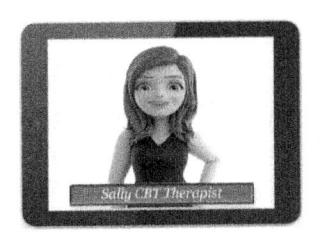

"So are you saying that our readers can actually grow and strengthen their pre-frontal cortex if they exercise it more?"

"Yes! That's the idea. It certainly looks like the more we use any part of the brain the stronger it gets."

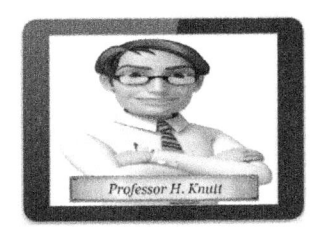

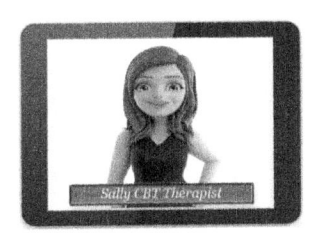

"Kate, do you have anything to add about self-observation?"

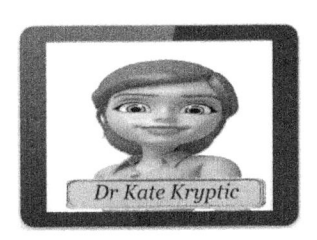

"I think self-observation is very important. I think Professor Knutt will agree that a fundamental aspect of any scientific approach is accurate observation. From a CBT perspective, standing back mentally and thinking about your own thinking processes will enable you to increase your awareness of your thoughts, feelings and behaviours, particularly when you are feeling distressed. This process of self-observation can assist you to become aware of the cycles that you engage in when you become emotional. I encourage my clients to take an exploratory approach to their problems and to think about their thinking processes. I usually suggest this because when my clients are able to think about their thinking or become curious about how think, they tend to feel less trapped by the content of their mind, and their minds automatic processes. They then have an opportunity to explore, to be curious and to notice their thoughts without judging themselves!!"

Chapter 8 – Further exploration

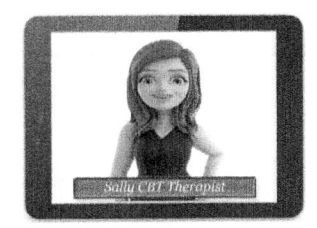

If you would like to look at an example of thoughts, feelings and behaviour sheets that people fill in when they have CBT, I have placed a few on the next number of pages and a blank sheet on the page overleaf. The example below will give you an idea of some of the types of things people write down and show their therapists. You can find out how to fill in these sheets in our other book "CBT Worksheets" or by talking to your therapist."

Example of Situation, thought, emotion and behaviour sheet

Situation	Thoughts (e.g., telling someone something that might hurt their feelings).	Emotion (e.g., feeling anxious) and reaction in body.	Behaviour (e.g., avoid the other person). How do others react to your behaviour?
Felt that a friend was trying to make me feel small	"She asked that question deliberately to try to undermine me"	Angry Irritated Feel agitated all over	Made an excuse to leave the situation for 5 minutes and then decided not to return at all. Others wondered where I was and perhaps thought I was acting oddly.
Not being invited to a colleagues wedding	She practically invited everyone else in the office apart from me. When she's got no one else to talk to she wants to be my friend."	Feel low and angry. I feel irritated being around her.	Ignore her whenever possible. Others start to think I am behaving oddly and ask me what's wrong. I just say everything's fine.

Thoughts, feelings & behaviour diary

Time: Date: Trigger situation:	Thoughts, e.g., "They must think that I'm an idiot?"	Emotion, e.g., anxiety, anger, shame, disgust	Behaviour, e.g., avoid situation

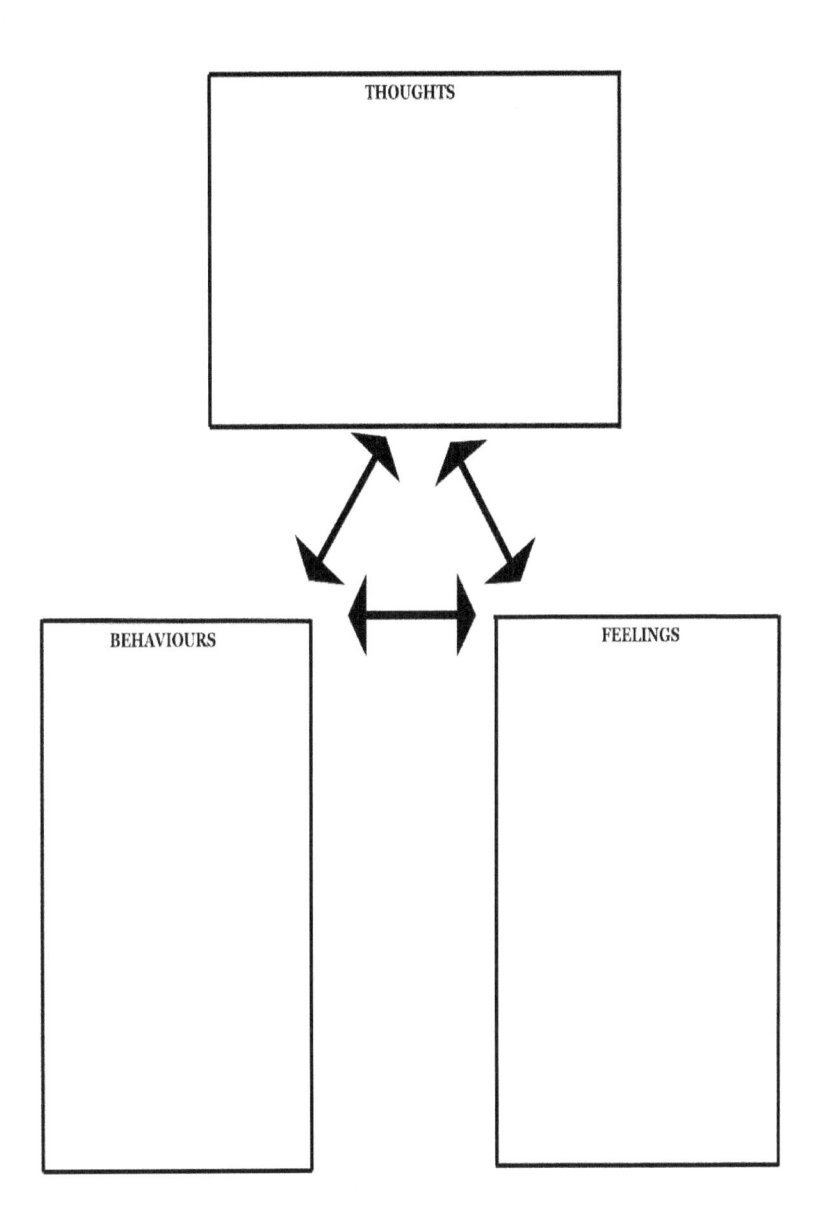

Standard thoughts, feelings, behaviour cycle

```
┌─────────────────────────┐
│        THOUGHTS         │
│                         │
│                         │
│                         │
└─────────────────────────┘
        ↕       ↕
┌──────────────┐   ┌──────────────┐
│  BEHAVIOURS  │↔  │   FEELINGS   │
│              │   │              │
│              │   │              │
│              │   │              │
└──────────────┘   └──────────────┘
```

Thoughts, physiology, emotion and behaviour diary

Automatic thoughts, e.g., "She doesn't like me"	Physiology, e.g., chest tightening	Emotion, e.g., anxiety	Behaviour, e.g., avoid contact with that person

Thought, physiology, emotion and behaviour sheet

Day:
Time:
Trigger situation:

Thoughts:

Physiological reactions

Emotion:

Behaviour:

Mood Diary

Please use this diary to keep a record of your mood. For each time period give yourself a score between 0 and 10 where 10 is the most that you can experience a feeling.

For the positive feeling box please rate how positive you felt during each time period as a whole. Examples of positivity may include, being interested, excited, enthusiastic, strong, proud etc.

For the negative feeling box please rate how negative you felt during the time period. Examples of negativity may include, feeling distressed, hostile, afraid, upset, ashamed and such like.

Day		Date	
Time period	Positive feeling 0 - 10	Negative feeling 0 - 10	
6am - 12pm			
12pm - 6pm			
6pm - 12am			

Day		Date	
Time period	Positive feeling 0 - 10	Negative feeling 0 - 10	
6am - 12pm			
12pm - 6pm			
6pm - 12am			

Day		Date	
Time period	Positive feeling 0 - 10	Negative feeling 0 - 10	
6am - 12pm			
12pm - 6pm			
6pm - 12am			

Day		Date	
Time period	Positive feeling 0 - 10	Negative feeling 0 - 10	
6am - 12pm			
12pm - 6pm			
6pm - 12am			

Day		Date	
Time period	Positive feeling 0 - 10	Negative feeling 0 - 10	
6am - 12pm			
12pm - 6pm			
6pm - 12am			

Day		Date	
Time period	Positive feeling 0 - 10	Negative feeling 0 - 10	
6am - 12pm			
12pm - 6pm			
6pm - 12am			

Day		Date	
Time period	Positive feeling 0 - 10	Negative feeling 0 - 10	
6am - 12pm			
12pm - 6pm			
6pm - 12am			

Chapter 9

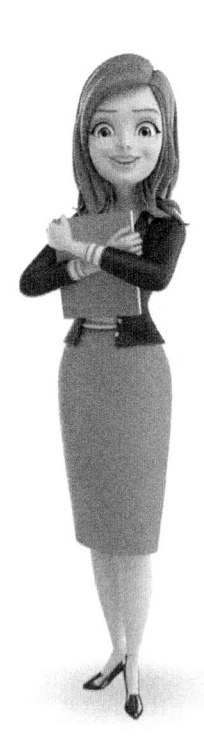

Cognitive Distortions

"We learned in previous chapters from both Big Jim and Professor Knutt that when we become distressed the way that we think can also change. The way that we think can affect the way that we view the world, the way that we feel, and the way that we behave."

"Can I ask you all to give your thoughts on cognitive distortions for our readers?

"I have just looked through some CBT texts, Sally and have found that cognitive distortions are included in most CBT books. High levels of distress can distort our perception, mood and behaviour, directly affecting the way we make sense of things. Our thinking style can move from being balanced, flexible, expansive, and considering to a more rigid style, not dissimilar to that you might expect of small children."

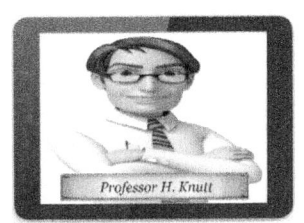

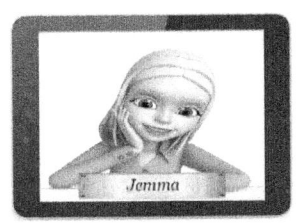

"I learned about cognitive distortions when I had CBT. It's a bit like somebody gives you some glasses, except you don't realise you're wearing them, and the glasses stop you seeing things straight. The glasses can make things seem much bigger or smaller than they really are."

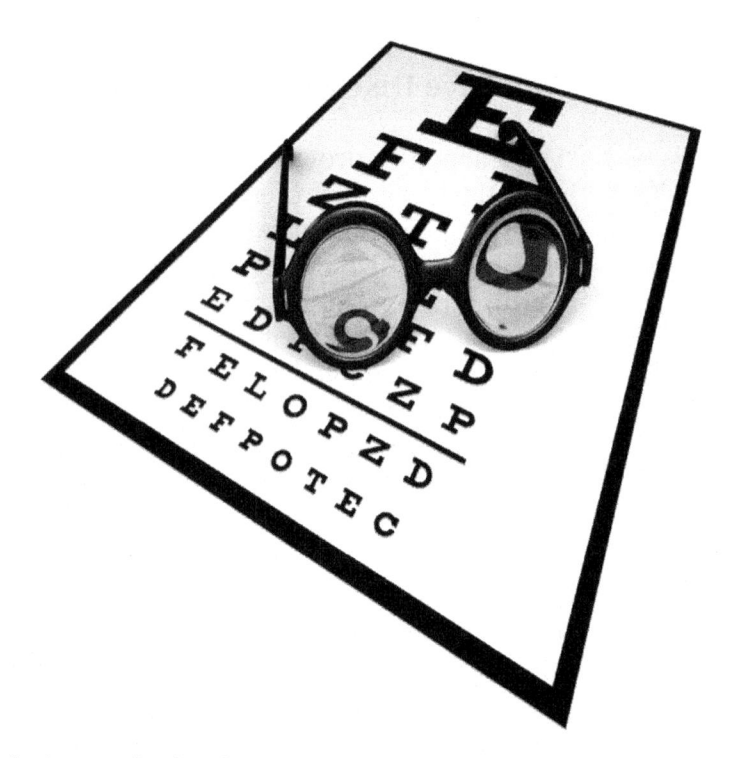

"It's worth checking that you're seeing things clearly and not seeing things as much bigger than they really are."

"When I began work with my therapist she helped me realise that when I got upset I didn't always see the world that clearly. Sometimes I filtered information so that I only saw what my mind would let me see. This meant I had a limited viewpoint and could not see what was really happening!"

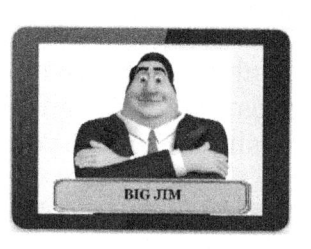

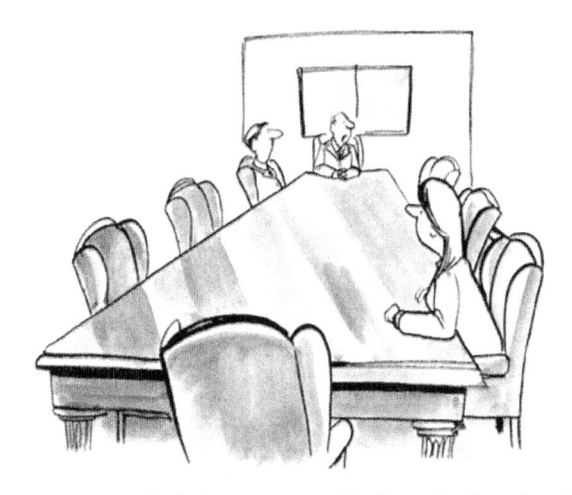

"I'm so glad that you could all make it today"

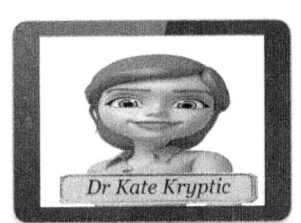

Dr Kate Kryptic

"When we become emotionally distressed we often may experience distortions in our thinking. In certain states we may think that we can see the future."

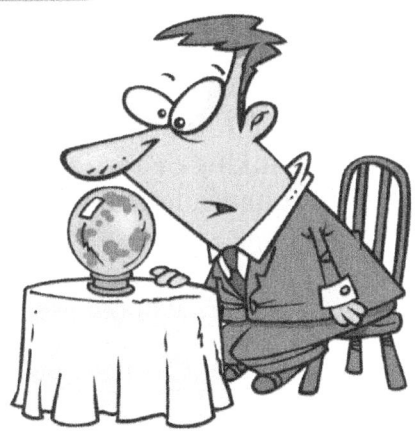

"Looks like it's going to be terrible tonight! I think I had better stay in."

"Or we can make things much bigger or smaller than they really are. Our cognitive distortions make our world appear like it is a very dangerous place to live in.

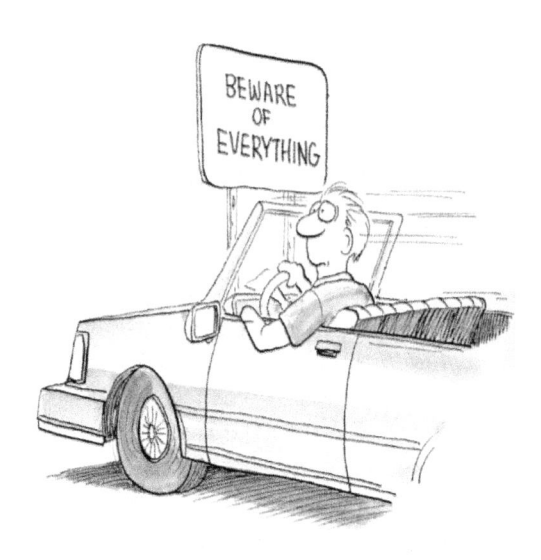

"I find it is vital in my work to help my clients to recognise when cognitive distortions are occurring so that as time progresses they can learn how to detach from that way of thinking. I have placed a table of some of the more common thinking distortions towards the end of this chapter for our readers to have a look at."

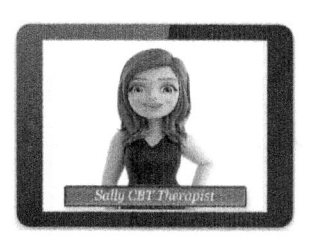

"Kate, how do you think our readers will benefit from noticing their cognitive distortions and then detaching from them?"

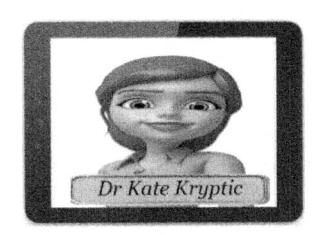

"I usually have a speech ready to tell my clients. It goes something like this - The moment we say to ourselves "Nothing ever works for me," "He or she always does that to me" or "I'm never considered," this will become our reality at that moment in time. If it were in fact true that nothing ever worked out, that all people always behave like this to us, all of the time, and that we were never considered, that indeed would be a pretty despairing place to be. Instead, how about if we choose to have awareness, without judgement of our thinking style? This will allow us to quickly acknowledge obvious distortions. This acknowledgement alone can have a marked positive impact on how we feel."

"I just think it is much more refreshing for people to be able to stand back from seeing the "alls" and "everythings" as facts and notice them instead as a thinking biases or styles."

Kate's table of thinking biases.

Thinking bias	What to look out for
All or nothing thinking	Viewing things as either right or wrong. There is no middle ground. Things are either perfect or fundamentally flawed. There is just black or white, grey does not exist, e.g., always/never, good/bad.
Disqualifying the positive	Positives don't count, there is nothing special about the way I did it, e.g., "That only happened because I was lucky."
Emotional reasoning	Using emotions as evidence, e.g., "I feel it, so it must be true."
Fortune telling	Predicting the future in a negative way without any real evidence, e.g., "It's going to be terrible."... "It will be a disaster"... "I just know it."
Mind reading	Drawing conclusions about what others are thinking without any evidence. "She doesn't like me."..."They think I am stupid."
Mental filtering	Selecting specific negative ideas to dwell on and ignoring all of the positive ones.
Should's, ought's & must's	Having ideas that things can only be done one way. "People should ..." "I must ..." "I really ought to ..." "He shouldn't have ..."
Personalising	Focusing on things in the immediate environment and connecting it to the self. Thinking for example, "she did that deliberately because she knew that I wouldn't like that!" The world revolves around the self.
Over-generalising	Taking single events or circumstances and viewing them as happening more often than they really do. Thinking that things happen everywhere.
Magnification or minimisation	Taking events and distorting them. Not dissimilar to looking at one's self through a fairground distorting mirror. Making things bigger or smaller than they really are.

Chapter 10

Rules

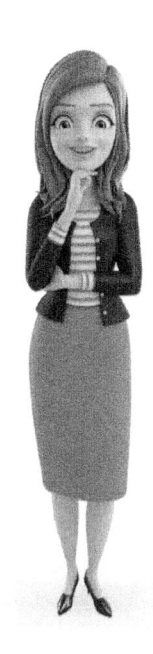

"When many people work with their CBT therapist, they find that their therapist helps them to identify the types of rules that they hold. We all live by rules and most of the time our rules help us. They work automatically in the background of our minds guiding us through cultural conventions and social occasions. We have literally hundreds of rules that guide our behaviour, for example, rules about queuing up, driving a car, attending a dinner party, how to use a knife and fork, what clothing to wear on what occasion etc. Most of the time we are completely unaware of our rules unless someone breaks them, for example, if somebody pushes in front of us in a queue, talks out loud in church and such like."

"Many of us also have rules that we use to protect ourselves from our deepest fears about ourselves, for example, "If I do everything right and make no mistakes, then I will be OK."

"So Big Jim did your therapist help you to identify any of your rules?"

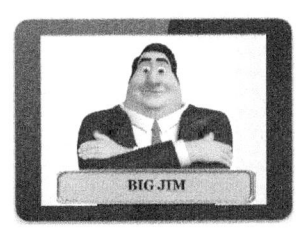

"Yes she did. My rules were mainly about how I wanted others to perceive me. They were a bit of a surprise to me when she helped me notice them. I kind of knew they were there in the background but hadn't really thought about them in that way before. They were something along the lines of "If I produce results and I am contributing then I will be OK." And, "If I meet the highest standards then I will be OK." My rules meant that I spent most of my time working and not spending time with my family. If I wasn't working I felt as though something wasn't quite right. I found it difficult to stop and rest even for five minutes. If I stopped working I felt guilty or anxious. It felt wrong if I wasn't achieving something."

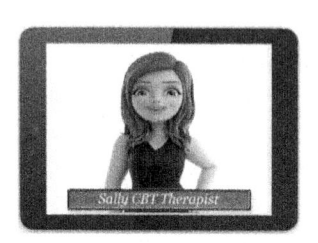

"So what impact did your rules have on your emotional wellbeing, and your family?"

"At the time I had taken on a difficult role at work. I worked and worked until eventually I became exhausted. When I wasn't able to work the way I did before I felt guilty about not working and started beating myself up over it. My wife told me I was neglecting her and that she would leave me if I didn't get help, and my children said that I didn't spend any time with them. When I thought about what was happening in therapy it really brought what I was doing to my attention. I thought I was doing all the extra work to help my family but obviously it didn't feel that way to them."

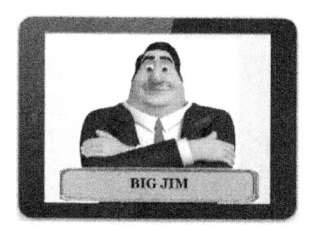

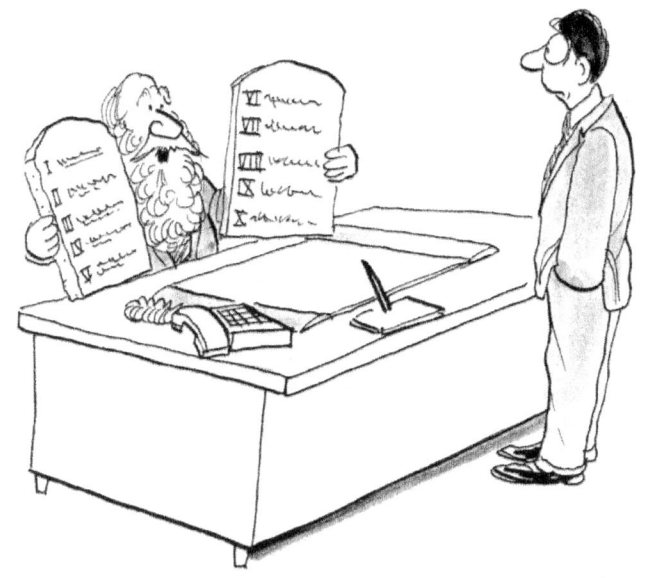

"Thanks for coming to see me to talk about new products. I couldn't help noticing that you like rules so I made you these."

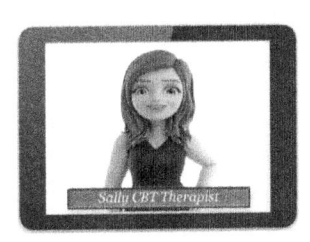

"I can see how these rules could have left you feeling quite stuck Big Jim!" "Do you have any experiences of rules in action Kate?"

"Last month a lady called Joan came to see me for an assessment. She was an attractive married lady in her early fifties who worked as a personal assistant to a European Chief Executive Officer of a multi-national company. When I spoke to Joan on the telephone to arrange her assessment appointment she told me she could only come for an assessment in the evening after work. She hinted that an appointment with myself was

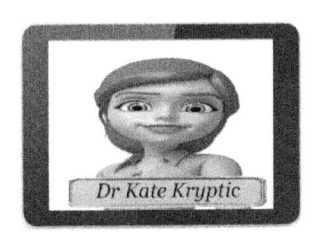

103

inconvenient for her and she was only really meeting me because her Psychiatrist has asked her to."

"Early in our meeting Joan told me how tired she felt and asked me when the assessment was going to end. Joan then dropped the bombshell that she was sure that therapy wasn't going to work for her and she was only really giving it a go because she wanted her Psychiatrist to be happy with her. She told me that she had been feeling fatigued for about two months and over the past number of weeks she had begun to work longer hours and was beginning to feel exhausted by it. I asked her what had led to her increased work hours and she told me that this was because she didn't feel as settled in her job as before and thought she needed to do extra work as her manger worked long hours and he might expect the same from her."

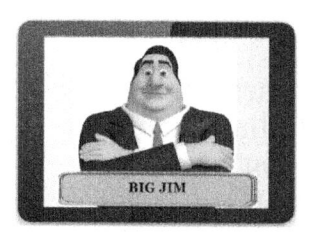

"Something else must have changed in her life!"

BIG JIM

"I did ask Joan about what had changed in the last couple of months and the only real change in her life was that her old boss Peter had moved divisions, and she now had a new young boss called Michael. Joan said that Michael was a good hard working manager and that she did not have any problems with him. When I enquired further it appeared that the main differences between her two managers, was that her old manager had given her lots of praise and reassurance for her work whereas her new manager just got on with his job and just left her to get

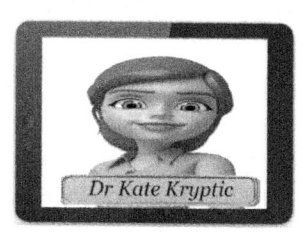

Dr Kate Kryptic

104

on with hers in a similar fashion. Essentially, the upshot was Michael didn't manage Joan at an emotional level. Michael's salary had a huge bonus component and he was working longer hours to enhance his wages, whereas Joan's wage was the same regardless of the hours that she worked. Joan didn't want to ask her new manager if everything was OK with her work as she thought that this may leave her looking weak and needy. As a result of this she said that she felt that she was never sure quite where she stood."

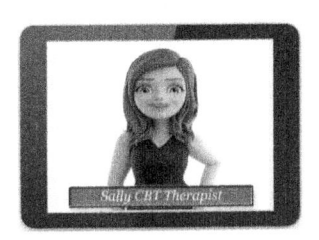

"So how did her rules influence what was happening?"

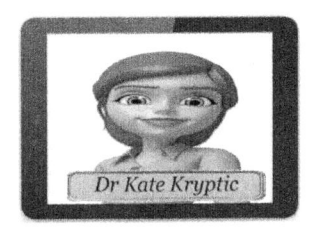

"As we discussed Joan's difficulties further, Joan was able to identify tension in her body as she talked about specific areas of her work. Using this tension we were able to identify two of her rules which turned out to be - "If people are happy with me and appreciate me at all times then I will be OK" and "If I feel strong and in control of my emotions at all times then I will be OK." It appeared that the lack of obvious appreciation from Michael for her work, and Joan not really wanting to talk with Michael about her work performance had gradually begun to break her rules about others being happy with her and appreciating her. The violation of this rule alongside her other rule about being in control of her feelings had led to her over-controlling her emotions and hiding her sense of vulnerability. My hypothesis was that these factors working together had led Joan to become depressed. Joan's symptoms of depression and her concentration difficulties in particular were worrying her as she feared this could lead to her making mistakes and then losing her job. Joan went on to explain that she did not have children and to a large extent her work and her husband had become her life and the thought of losing her job made her feel suicidal."

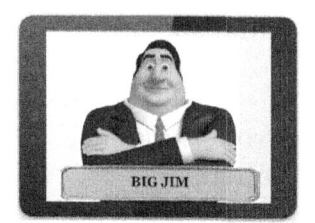

BIG JIM

"Excuse me butting in here but it sounds like Joan didn't realise that she had begun to start digging a big hole for herself!"

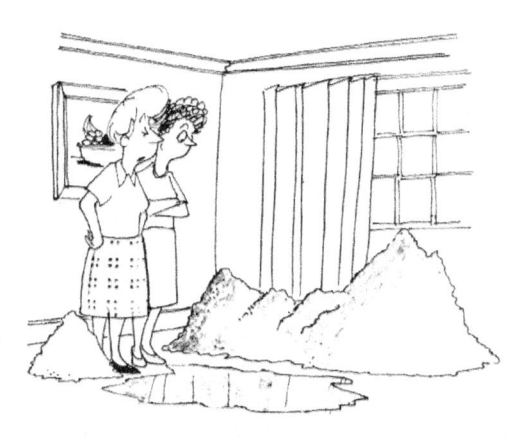

"Has anyone asked Joan what she's doing down there?"

"Exactly! Joan was by now on the verge of visiting her General Practitioner to ask for a sickness certificate, which would probably mean that she would be signed off from work for weeks. It appeared that Joan had worked her way into a situation where she had the potential to dig herself deeper and

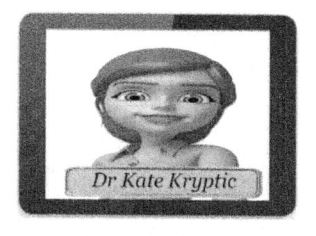

Dr Kate Kryptic

deeper into a depressive position with increased rule violations still to come."

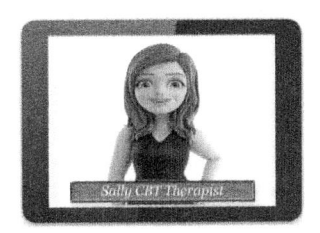

"I guess to an outsider the solution to Joan's problem is quite obvious!"

"Yes Sally! You know as well as me how difficult it is to see things logically when you are in a hole. A natural tendency is to want to keep digging. Of course, we know that Joan would need to allow herself to be vulnerable, talk to her manager about her struggles coping, reduce her working hours to normal levels and ask for regular reviews of her work from Michael. These obvious solutions as you might expect would not have felt right to Joan due to the rigidity of her rules. Her main focus was on blaming herself and telling herself that it was her fault. Her sense of wellbeing was completely dependent on somebody else praising her.

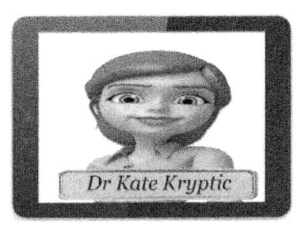

"Essentially, the main message that I try to get across to clients is that rules are developed by our brains to keep us safe. They are usually created early in our lives as children. They may help us during that period of time. However, as we grow older, rules can become out of date and **maladaptive**. By maladaptive I mean the rules hold her back rather than working for her"

"So are you saying that Joan's rule "If people are happy with me and appreciate me at all times then I'll be OK" may have helped her as a child?

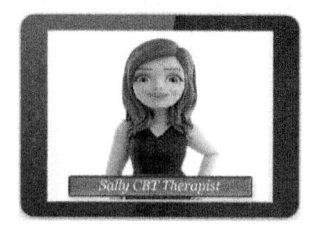

"Yes, the rule may have helped her with her teachers at school or even with her parents. But when she was working for her new manager this old rule started to become very unhelpful."

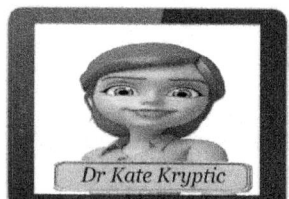

Chapter 10 – Further exploration

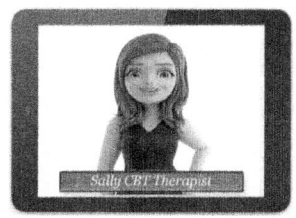

If you would like to investigate what your rules are, begin by writing a list of what you expect from yourself and others. The belief rule challenging exercises that we have included are designed to bring the impact of your rules into your awareness. This exercise is not powerful enough on its own to change your rules, but it may make your rules slightly more malleable/flexible. It is usually a good idea to talk through what your rules are with your therapist. More user friendly versions of these forms can be found in our book "CBT Worksheets".

My Rule Sheet

For example, If I am strong and in control, then I will be OK

If I am..
then I will be OK

If I am..
then I will be OK

If I am..
then I will be OK

If I am..
then I will be OK

If I am..
then I will be OK

My Rule Sheet

For example, If others like me at all times then I will be OK

If others..
then I will be OK

If others..
then I will be OK

If others ....
then I will be OK

If others..
then I will be OK

If others..
then I will be OK

Rule challenging exercise

| Rule | How old is your rule? | If you gave yourself an opportunity to have another rule, what rule would you pick? |

How real and familiar does your rule feel?

Where do you think your rule came from?

What impact does your rule have on your life?

How do you think you might feel if you choose to live by your new rule as much as you did the old one?

If you learnt your rule from a person where do you think he or she learnt it from?

What benefits does your rule have on your life?

How does knowing that you can choose to have another rule make you feel?

Do you want to keep your rule?

Were you born with your rule?

Chapter 11

Limiting Beliefs

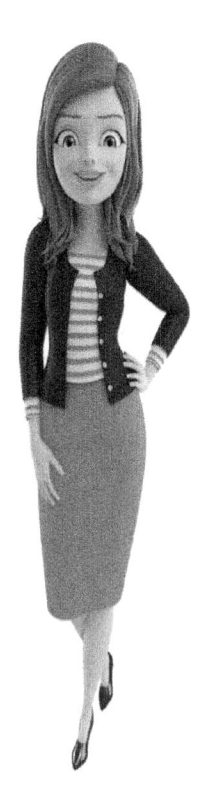

"Generally speaking, limiting beliefs are deeply held ideas about ourselves that we fear might be true. By the time that we become adults, these beliefs can become so set within us, that we feel that they are part of us. Sometimes we hold them so deeply, that we have forgotten what they are. We may also carry out numerous 'safety behaviours' to protect ourselves from them without being aware of it. Most of us do not realise that they are running us."

"So Big Jim. Did your therapist help you identify any of your limiting beliefs?"

"Yes, she did. I discovered that one of my limiting beliefs was "I am a failure!"… "The funny thing about it was no matter how hard I worked or how much I achieved the belief "I am a failure" was always still there. It seemed like what I had done in the past counted for nothing. Trying to prove the belief wrong demanded so much of my time that it affected my health, and the happiness of my family. I didn't realise it was driving me so much. I didn't feel in control of my life. It drove me to do more and more. I didn't really know how to stop!"

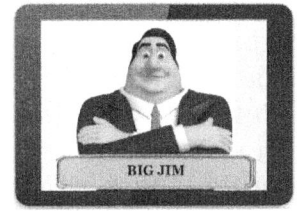

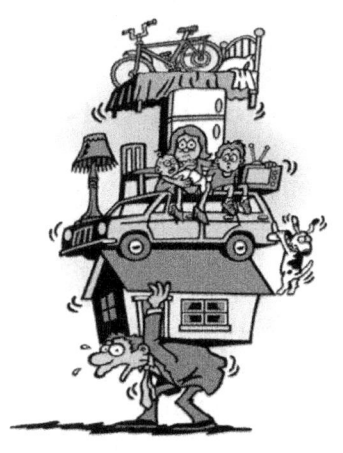

"Jim dear! Do you think you might be trying to do too much?"

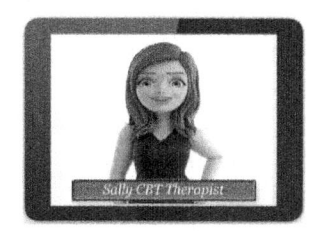

"That must have been terribly difficult for you! How did you find out it was there?"

"My therapist helped me to notice that in many situations I was experiencing high levels of painful emotions that were inconsistent with the situation that I faced with. For example, we identified that I had an over the top reaction to even small amounts of criticism. After this she helped me recognise that the belief "I am a failure" was the main driver for my emotional reaction. This emotional reaction was the primitive part of my brain trying to protect me from being a failure. After I became aware of this, if I noticed my emotions were too extreme or I felt I wanted to over-react in any situation, I usually took a minute out to see if a limiting belief was influencing me."

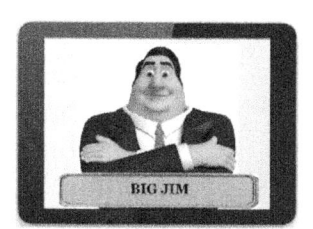

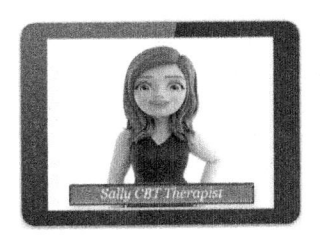

"Professor Knutt, is there are any scientific evidence behind the development of limiting beliefs, because we are obviously not born believing these types of things about ourselves!"

"Well the most obvious way to develop limiting beliefs does not really need any scientific evidence or scientific explanation. If parents or caregivers tell their children that they are stupid, worthless, or a failure this can lead to their children developing limiting beliefs! Equally if parents or caregiver treat their children in a poor way this can lead to the development of limiting beliefs!"

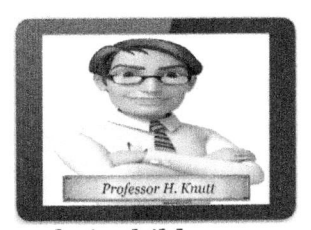

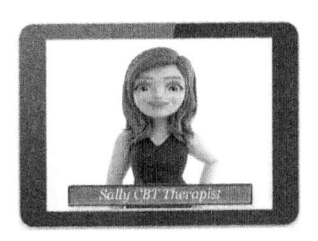

"Are there other ways that people develop beliefs? Perhaps ways they might not normally think about? I am saying this because many of my clients have not had abusive parents in their childhood but yet they still have limiting beliefs. Perhaps if you could give just one or two suggestions to give our readers some ideas about how this might work."

"There are lots of theoretical suggestions, but I'll need to set the scene first so that you will understand my reasoning. In 2014, researchers from the University of Michigan Jacek Debiec and Regina Sullivan completed some interesting research on rats. They taught young female rats to fear the smell of peppermint by pairing the smell of

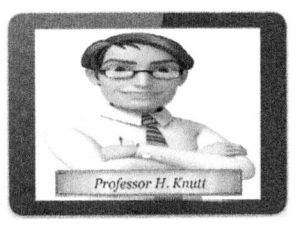

115

peppermint with electric shocks. The female rats then became pregnant and gave birth. After the mothers had given birth experimenters re-exposed the mother rats to the peppermint smell again while they were with their babies. The researchers found that infant rats learned to fear the peppermint smell by noticing the scent of fear given off by their mother. Brain scans carried out of the baby rats revealed that a fear of peppermint was programed directly into infant rats' amygdala. As we talked about earlier the amygdala is the seat of our natural response to threat. There is growing evidence that infant children's brains operate in the same way as baby rats, both in the womb and after birth up until the age of 6 months. Research is still being carried out right now at this moment."

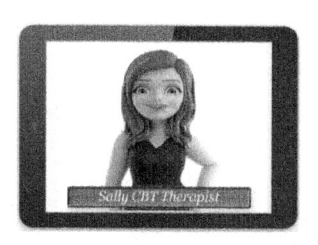

"Sorry, Professor Knutt, I don't quite get what this has to do with beliefs?

"I think what Professor Knutt is saying is that children basically absorb their parents' fears."

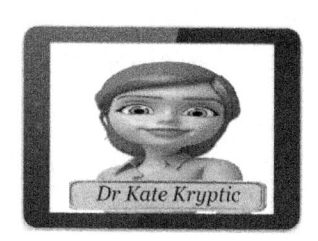

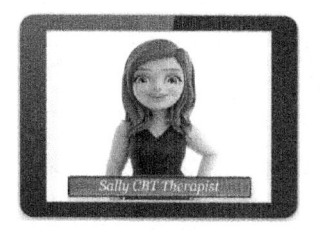

"So Professor Knutt are you saying that Big Jim learned his fear of failure from one of his parents somehow?"

"It is a bit of a stretch theoretically, but yes that is really what I am saying! The implication is that there is a possibility that we are biologically preprogramed to accept a rapid transfer of information from our parents. In fact, the reason why Jacek Debiec set up his experiments in the first place was because he had come across many people who were presenting with nightmares and post-trauma symptoms connected to the Holocaust in World War II. The issue that confused him most of all was that these particular adults with post-trauma symptoms had not even been born during the Holocaust. They were children of survivors of the Holocaust and somehow and someway they had taken on the fears of their parents."

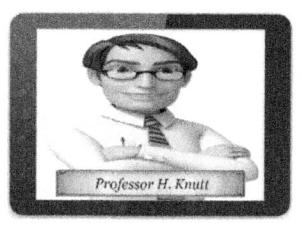

"However, this is not the only way that we can develop belief systems. There is also a process called social learning that we could consider."

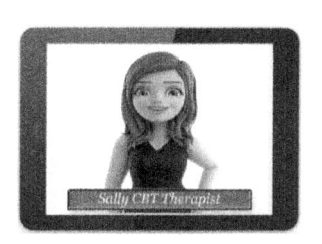

"Can you tell us more about this?"

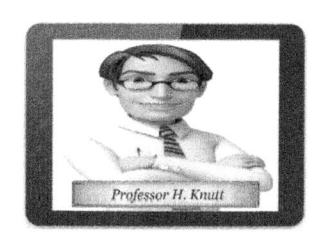

"In 1977, Albert Bandura wrote about a process he identified in children called observational learning which is now known as social learning theory. He witnessed that children act as little information processers watching and copying the behaviour of important others, or role models. If for example, Big Jim's father felt that he needed to do things perfectly and to high standards, Big Jim may have learnt this way of behaving from his father. Equally, he could have learnt it from his mother."

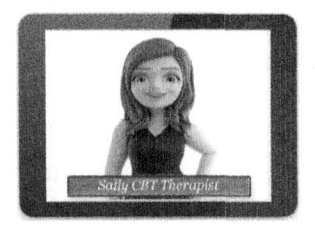

"Kate, would you be able to explain for our readers how Cognitive Therapists sometimes go about identify limiting beliefs?"

"Therapists will usually start off with a situation where their client have quite intense emotion. Clients determine if their emotion is more intense than they think is appropriate for the situation. Therapists then help their clients complete something called a **downward arrow** exercise. With a downward arrow exercise therapists help their clients to keep following feelings and thoughts until their client reaches the deepest fears that they hold about themselves. I have put an example of a downward arrow exercise on the next page."

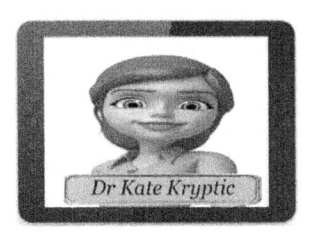

Therapist starts with painful thought associated with intense emotion.
"Why does this keep happening to me?"

Therapist draws attention to the client's body and asks about emotional reaction to having thought (e.g., stomach tightening, fists clenching etc.)

"Feel low, deflated"

Therapist then asks – "If this thought were true what would this say about you"
"That I'm stupid!"

Therapist asks client to note feelings in body when client has thought "That I'm stupid!"

"Embarrassed ashamed"

Therapist then asks – "If this thought were true what would this say about you"
"There is something wrong with me!"

Therapist repeats as above.

"Embarrassed ashamed"

Therapist then asks – "If this thought were true what would this say about you"
"I'm pathetic, useless"

Therapist repeats as above.

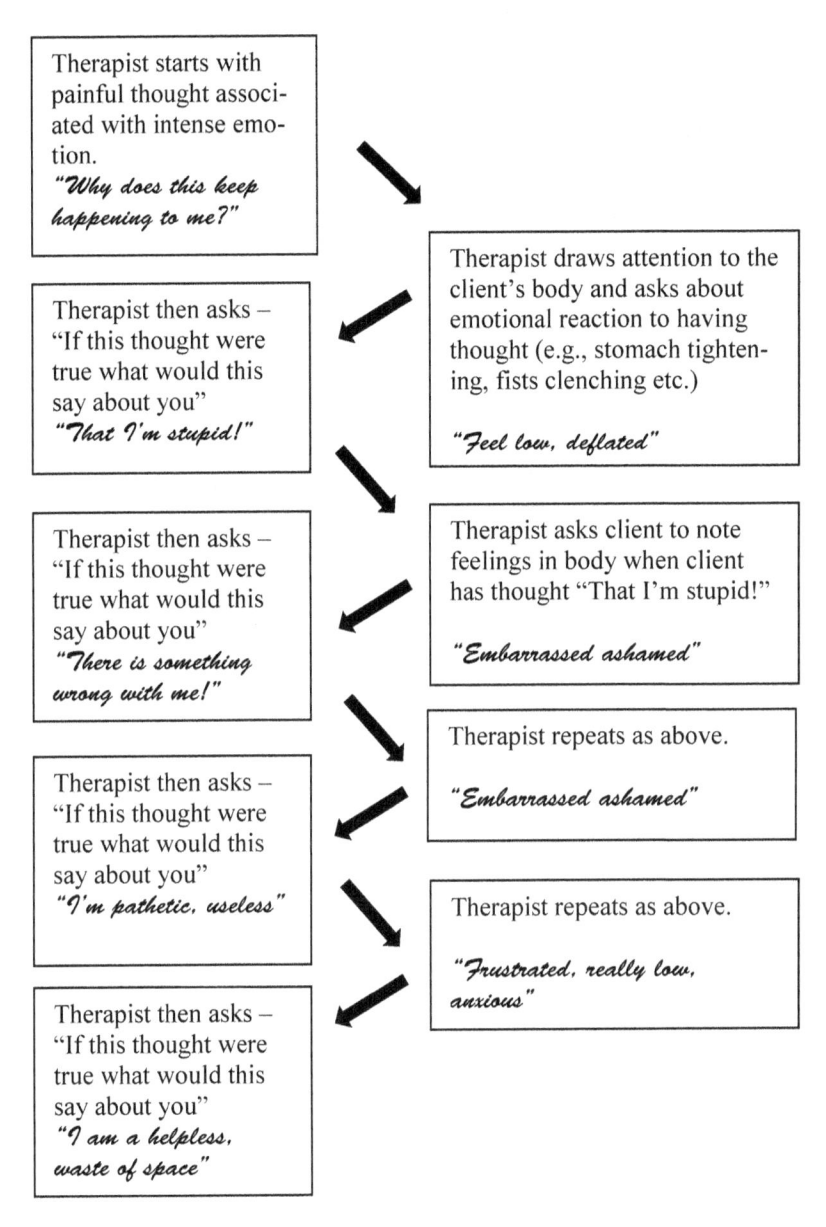

"Frustrated, really low, anxious"

Therapist then asks – "If this thought were true what would this say about you"
"I am a helpless, waste of space"

Kate's downward arrow example

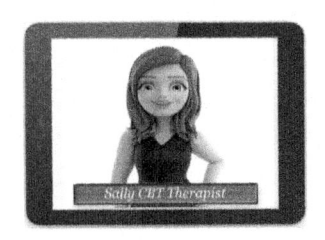

"Are there any other exercises that CBT therapists might use to help people explore their beliefs?"

"Yes, several. The types of exercises used will be dependent on the skill, experience and training of the therapist. At the most simple level the therapist will draw attention to the client's belief system and ask questions about it. Big Jim would you mind taking yourself back to when you were a client having CBT so that I demonstrate a simple exercise with you for our readers?

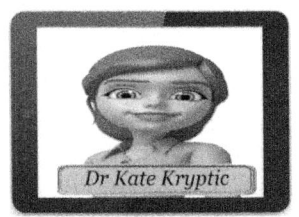

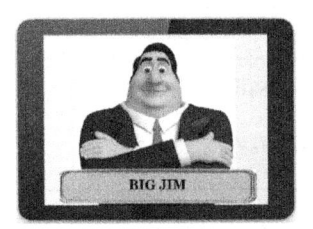

"Yes...Sure!"

"If we start with your unhelpful belief "I am a failure!" How real and familiar does that belief seem to you?"

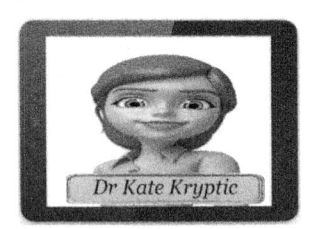

120

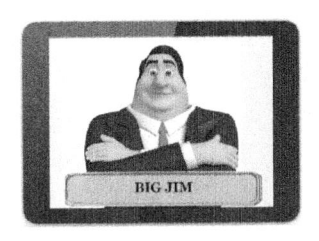

Big Jim: "It feels real when I'm in it! It seems that it's been there for as long as I can remember."

Dr Kate Kryptic: "What impact does the belief 'I am a failure' have on your life?"

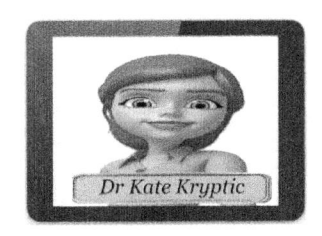

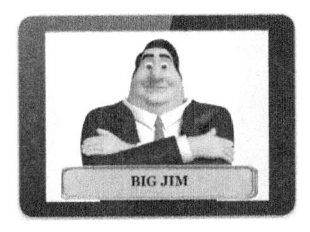

Big Jim: "It makes me feel rubbish and inferior a lot of the time and continues to affect my self-esteem."

Dr Kate Kryptic: "What benefits has the belief 'I am a failure' had on your life?"

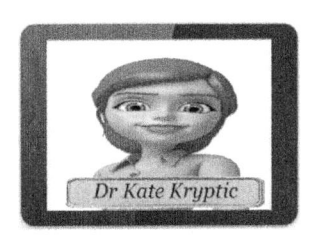

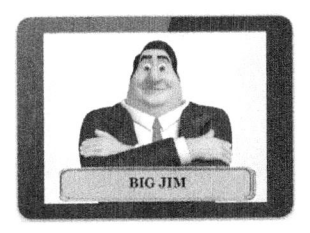

Big Jim: "I think it has helped me achieve some things that I might not have done. But, then again, I have never really celebrated my achievements, just moved onto the next one!"

"When you were a new born baby did you believe I am a failure?"

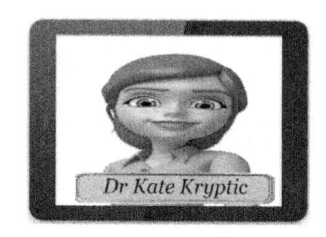

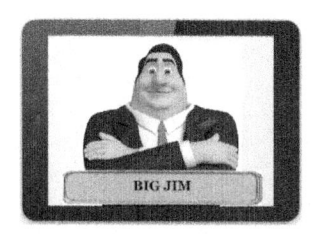

— Dr Kate Kryptic

"Of course I didn't!"

— BIG JIM

"How old is the belief I am a failure would you say?"

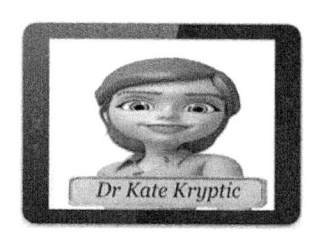

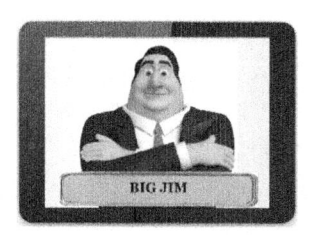

— Dr Kate Kryptic

"I guess it's about 30 old!"

— BIG JIM

"Where do you think it came from?"

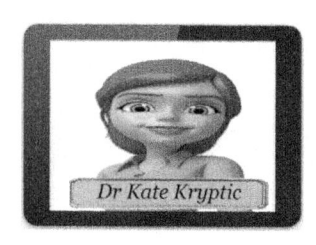

— Dr Kate Kryptic

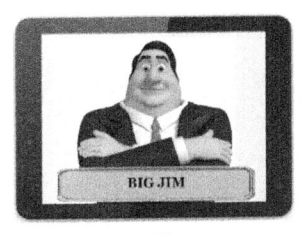

Big Jim: "I think I learnt it when I was young from my mother. When I was little, learning to do maths, draw and create things. There was always some improvement that she thought I could make in some way!"

Dr Kate Kryptic: "What might your mother have believed about herself would you say?"

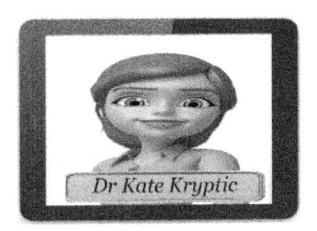

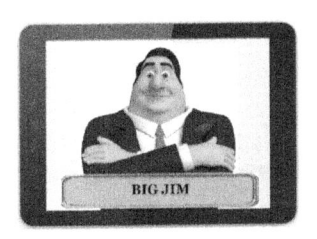

Big Jim: "She probably believed that she was a failure as well. That's more than likely why she wanted me to do so well at school."

Dr Kate Kryptic: "Where do you think that she learnt to believe that she was a failure?"

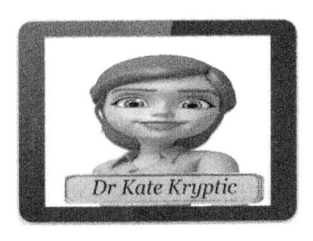

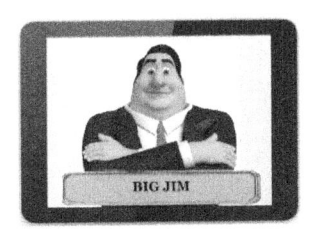

Big Jim: "She probably learnt it from her parents I would guess. I know her father struggled particularly with his upbringing."

"Do you want to keep the belief - I am a failure?"

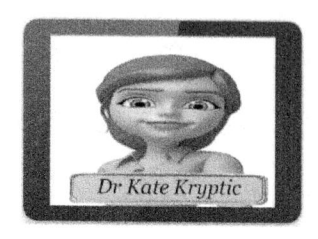

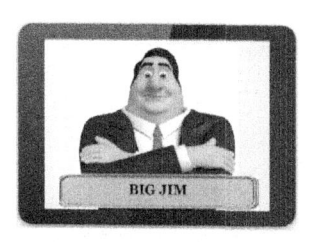

Dr Kate Kryptic

"Not any more. No!"

BIG JIM

"So if you gave yourself an opportunity to believe something else about yourself right now, what type of belief would you pick?"

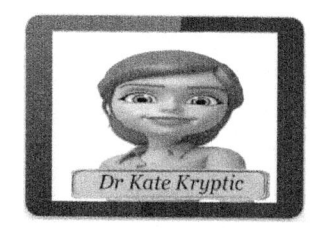

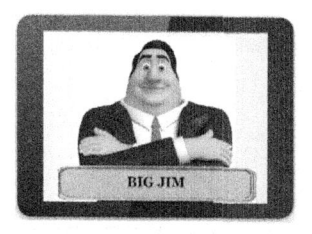

Dr Kate Kryptic

"That I really am OK, just as I am!"

BIG JIM

"How do you think you might feel if you choose to believe that belief as much as your old unhelpful belief from the past?"

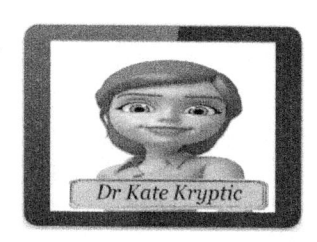

Dr Kate Kryptic

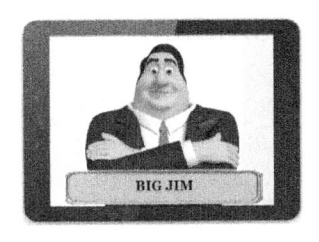

"Relieved, I wouldn't feel that I needed to do quite so much. I could be the same as everybody else."

"How does knowing that you can choose to believe something else about yourself make you feel?"

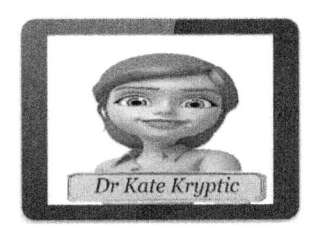

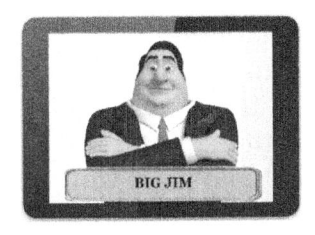

"I feel more in charge of my life. I guess!"

"That's great. Thanks very much for helping our readers with that exercise Big Jim. I know you've engaged with CBT and I appreciate your help in demonstrating the exercise. I often find it more difficult with clients in practice. I think it's very important for us all to know what limiting beliefs we may have. If we don't there is a high probability that rules and expectations connected to them will be running our lives without us even realising it."

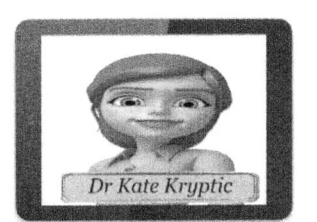

Chapter 11 – Further exploration

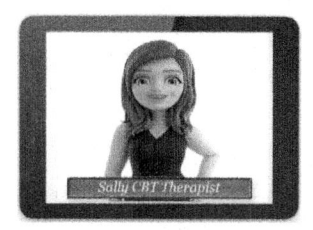

Core beliefs are very difficult to challenge and it is highly likely that part of you will cling onto them tightly. Beliefs can feel like fixed truths and it often seems like they simply cannot be contested. Many of us spend huge amounts of our time, (perhaps even changing the way we live our lives), attempting to prove them wrong. We may also develop self-imposed rules about our behaviour in order to compensate against them.

Dropping our beliefs can feel quite frightening, as in most cases we will have devoted huge amounts of time and resources to compensating against them (trying to prove them wrong). Beliefs can feel as though they are part of us and sometimes we might feel that we might lose part of our identity without them. Beliefs have the power to impact on our relationships, our choice of partner and occupation. There are no areas of our lives that are untouched by our beliefs.

The belief exercises that follow are predominantly designed to bring your beliefs into awareness. These exercises are not powerful enough on their own to change or to destabilise beliefs, but they may make your beliefs more flexible.

The down ward arrow exercise

The downward arrow exercise is very difficult exercise to complete by yourself. It can produce high levels of emotional distress and will involve you accessing your deepest fears. Understandably, most people feel an aversion to completing a downward arrow exercise alone, and it is often easier to do it with a therapist.

To start the exercise bring a thoughts that troubles you often to your awareness. Scan your body while you hold this thought in awareness and notice the impact that your thought has on you at an emotional or physiological level.

Focussing on how you feel ask yourself – "If this thought were true what would it say or mean about me?" Repeat this questioning process with each progressive thought that your mind produces until you find yourself repeating earlier thoughts. When your thoughts become most painful or aversive you are likely to be accessing a belief. Beliefs are judgemental unconditional statements about the self or others beginning with the word I or others. For example, "I am bad" "I am worthless" "I am inadequate" "I am weak" "Others cannot be trusted"

Downward arrow exercise

- Start with thought connected to intense emotion
- Notice physiological reaction
- If this thought were true what would that say about me?
- Notice physiological reaction
- If this thought were true what would that mean about me?
- Notice physiological reaction
- If this thought were true what would that say about me?
- Notice physiological reaction
- Continue until you reach core belief. Use new sheet if necessary

Belief challenging exercise

| Belief | How old is your belief? | If you gave yourself an opportunity to believe something else, what belief would you pick? |

How real and familiar does your belief feel?

Where do you think your belief came from?

What impact does your belief have on your life?

How do you think you might feel if you choose to believe your new belief as much as the old one?

If you learnt a belief from a person where do you think he or she learnt it from?

What benefits does your belief have on your life?

How does knowing that you can choose to believe something else make you feel?

Do you want to keep your belief?

Were you born with your belief?

Chapter 12

Simple CBT cycles

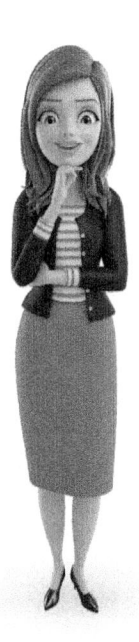

"Many CBT therapists draw out cycles to explain people's problems using their white boards. A general idea behind drawing out these cycles is to help people recognise that some of the things that they do can tend to keep their problems in place. Once you realise that you have a cycle in place, you will then need to work out how to break the cycle."

"There are several ways to draw out cycles. I'd like us to start by making a connection between beliefs, rules and safety behaviours. It is usually drawn out on a white board like this."

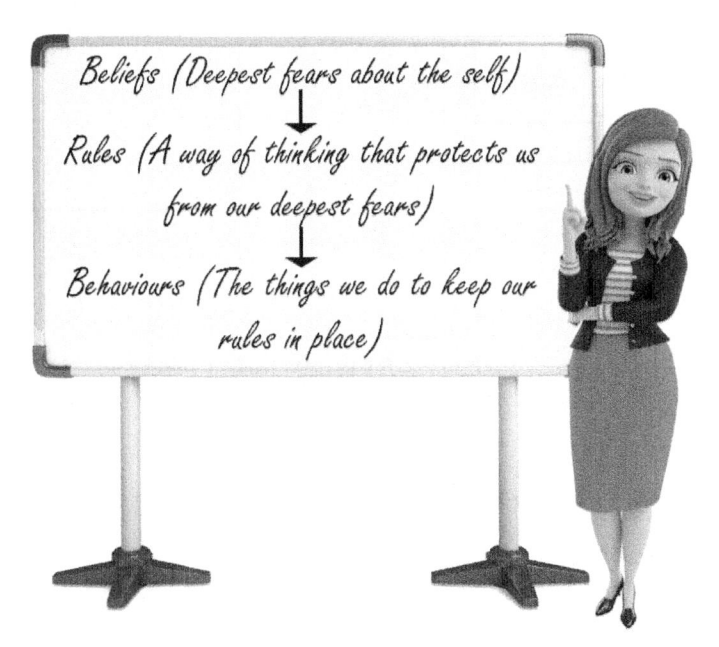

Beliefs (Deepest fears about the self)
↓
Rules (A way of thinking that protects us from our deepest fears)
↓
Behaviours (The things we do to keep our rules in place)

"It will makes much more sense however to see how this is drawn out in real life, however.... Big Jim, perhaps you and I could work on this for our readers ... If you don't mind?"

"That's fine with me!"

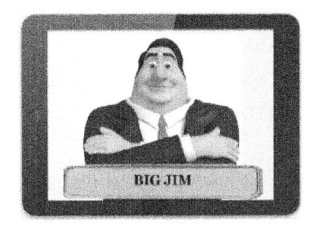

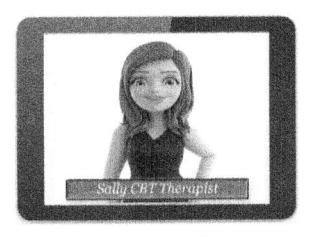

"Big Jim, our readers might remember that in Chapter 10 you mentioned that you had a belief "I am failure". You said that he felt driven to do more and more to prove it wrong. Can you remind me what you and your therapist decided what your rule was?"

"The rule I had was "If I am successful at all times and if people are happy with my work then I will be OK.""

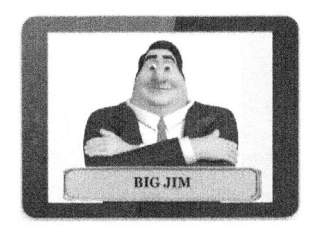

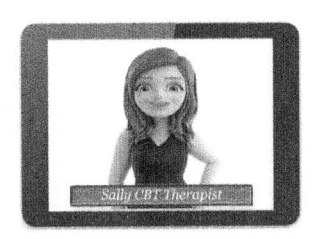

"And, what behaviours did you outline with your therapist that kept this rule in place?"

"The main things I did were to work very long hours, make sure everything I did everything perfectly, not take breaks, compare my work with others to make sure that I was the best, and get angry if anybody made suggestions about improvements."

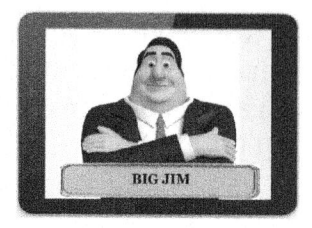

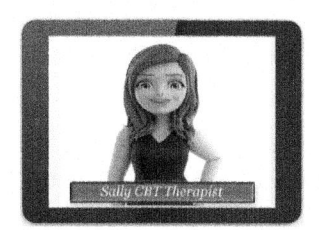

"Thanks Big Jim. I am now going to put these ideas into a diagram as you would have done with your therapist."

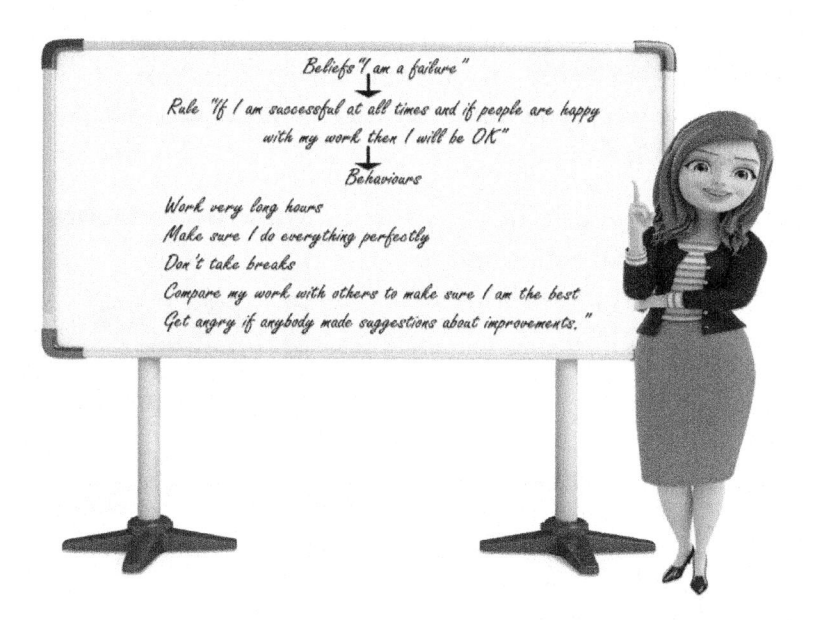

Beliefs "I am a failure"
↓
Rule "If I am successful at all times and if people are happy with my work then I will be OK"
↓
Behaviours

Work very long hours
Make sure I do everything perfectly
Don't take breaks
Compare my work with others to make sure I am the best
Get angry if anybody made suggestions about improvements."

"So Big Jim. How did you and your therapist turn this information into a cycle?"

132

"My therapist asked me what happened when I felt I could not keep to my rule of being successful at what I did at all times. I told her this made me feel highly anxious and on edge. We worked out that I was getting these feelings because my belief "I am a failure" was being activated when I was not maintaining my rule. When this happened I felt that I needed to do what I was doing before even more, to protect myself from my fear of failure. This led to me working even harder. Eventually, I worked so hard that I became ill and needed to be signed off work."

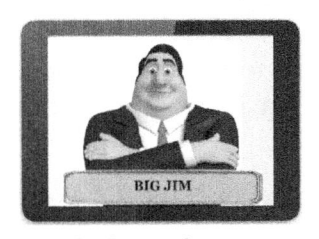

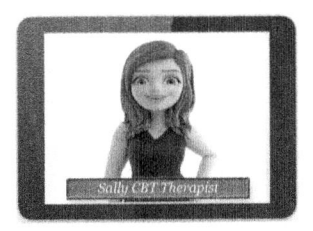

"How did your therapist help you recognise that you were getting involved in a cycle?"

"Well, she asked me about how my very best attempts at proving to myself that I wasn't a failure, may have actually ended up with me believing that I was a failure even more. It's a bit obvious when I think about it now because I'm not in it, but my wife was unhappy with me and my kids were upset because I was working so much. So I guess I could tell myself that I was failing as a husband and as a father. My boss was OK about me taking some time out, but I felt that I had let work down as they had to pay somebody else to come in to do my job for me. I just got myself into a bit of a mess with it all and felt that I was failing in all areas of my life."

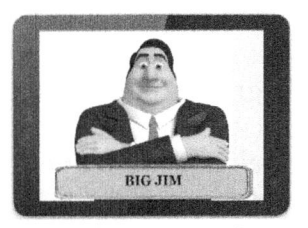

133

"My guess is that your therapist would have drawn something that might have looked a bit like the diagram I have put on my board."

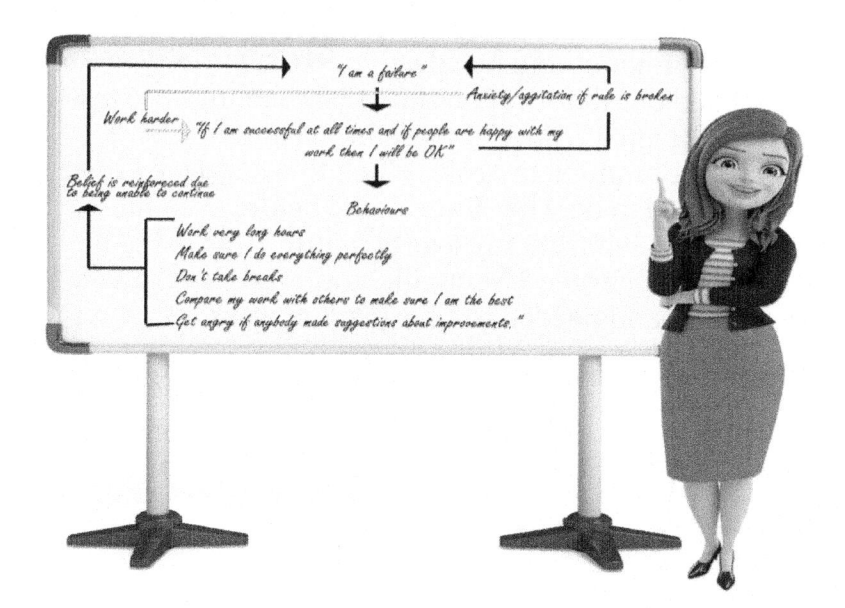

"Yes, that was similar to the diagram she wrote on her board. Once it was in front of me in black and white, I couldn't pretend to myself that it wasn't happening. It was then really obvious to me that I needed to break my cycle."

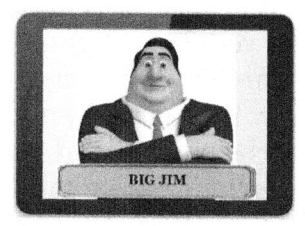

Other CBT cycles

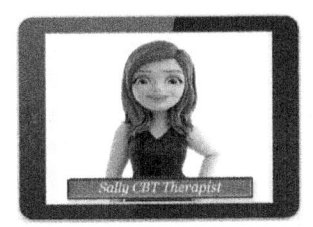

"The most common CBT cycle is a thoughts, feelings behaviour and physiology cycle, originally credited to a Psychologist called Christine Padesky. In this cycle, thoughts influence feelings, feelings influence behaviour, and behaviour reinforces thoughts. The whole thing works a bit like a vicious cycle."

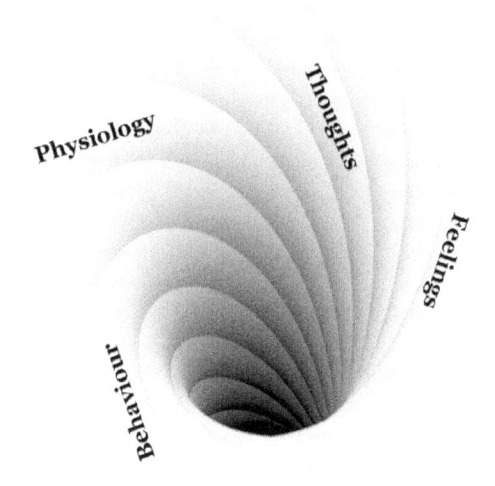

"I will give some examples as it will make a lot more sense that way."

"A few months ago I worked with a lady called Vera who had been depressed for a short while. She worried a lot

135

about what others thought of her and deep down inside she had fears that she was weak and incapable. She had a voluntary job in her local village shop for a couple of hours a week which had given her a lot of satisfaction previously. She had enjoyed this job in the past because it had been an opportunity for her to catch up with the local villagers and find out what has been going on in her neighbours' lives. On one particular day she was thinking about whether she might phone up and cancel her stint in the shop. She was thinking about this because she hasn't quite been herself due to her symptoms of depression and was concerned about what others might think of her. I have drawn her thoughts, feelings, physiology and behaviour cycle on the next page."

Feared meaning
I am weak
I am incapable

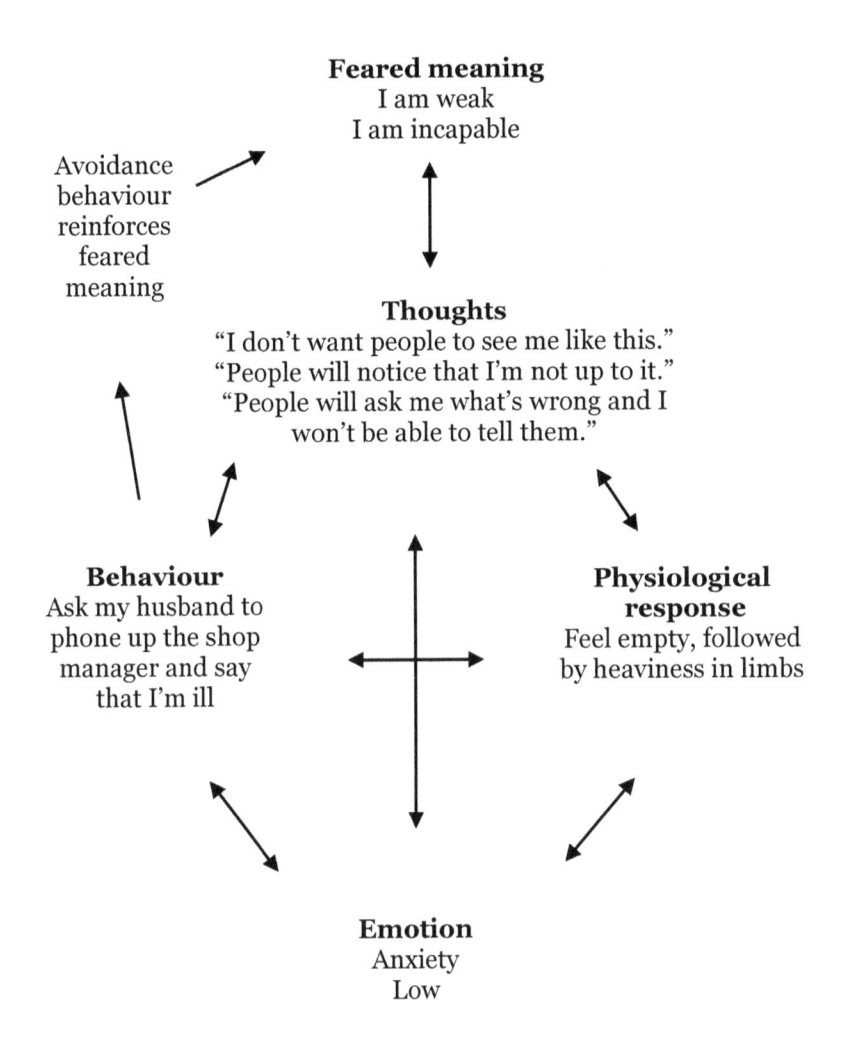

Avoidance behaviour reinforces feared meaning

Thoughts
"I don't want people to see me like this."
"People will notice that I'm not up to it."
"People will ask me what's wrong and I won't be able to tell them."

Behaviour
Ask my husband to phone up the shop manager and say that I'm ill

Physiological response
Feel empty, followed by heaviness in limbs

Emotion
Anxiety
Low

"I notice that in this diagram that most of the arrows are pointing in both directions. So where does it start?"

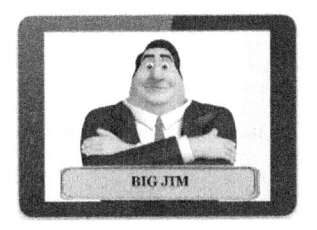

BIG JIM

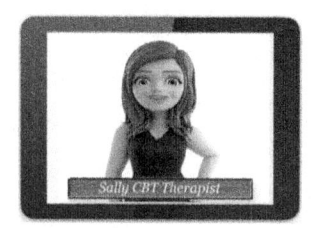

"The real starting point for Vera, which isn't in the diagram, is Vera looking at her calendar and noticing that she had a shift in the shop coming up. The cycle could then actually start with her physiological response, her emotions, her thoughts or an immediate reactive behaviour. The essence of the cycle is that each part of the cycle is needed to keep the cycle going."

"How many of these types of CBT cycles are there?"

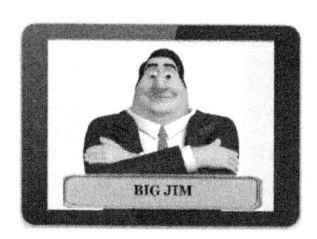

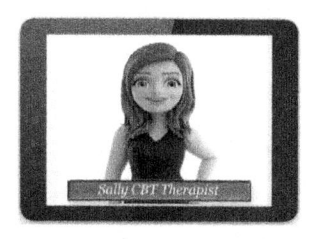

"There are a lot. Most of the major writers on CBT have identified cycles that relate to specific conditions. There are cycles for health anxiety, social anxiety, obsessional compulsive disorder, generalised anxiety disorder. In fact, all diagnosable mental health conditions now have CBT cycles dedicated to them. In many respects the diagrams are all very similar. I will put a selection of these cycles at the end of this chapter for our readers to look through. If our readers want to they can fill them in with their therapists. Information about how these cycles work is contain in our other book "CBT Worksheets."

"Once our readers have drawn out their cycle this will give them an idea about what they need to do next."

"A natural progression after identifying a cycle is to move onto creating goals. CBT has a strong emphasis on goals. I have put a typical goal sheet on the next page."

"I think many of our readers might be wondering where they might start when they want to break a cycle. What would you suggest to them?"

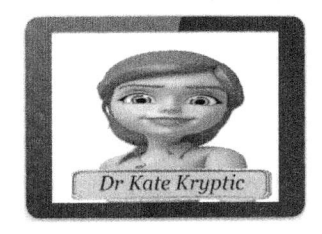

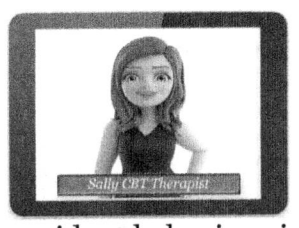

Dr Kate Kryptic

Sally CBT Therapist

"A cycle can be broken by directing attention to any one area of a cycle. This is because each part of a cycle is dependent on other parts of the cycle to keep it in place. For example, if avoidant behaviour is challenged this creates less opportunities to mull over negative thoughts. If feeling sad is soothed away there is less tendency to mull over negative thoughts. If negative thoughts are challenged or dampened there is less intense emotion. It is hard for the cycle to maintain itself if pieces of it are missing. Later on we will talk about breaking patters like this. As I just mentioned a natural progression once cycles are identified is to work on goals. I have put a completed goal sheet on the next page for our readers to look at.

Old Cycle

Beliefs
"I am incompetent"
"I am not likeable"
"I am insignificant"

Old rule - If am in control of my environment at all times then I wil be OK

Old rule - If others like me at all times then I wil be OK

Old rule - If am in control of my feelings at all times then I wil be OK

Old rule - If others notice my achievements at all times then I wil be OK

Old behaviours used to keep rule in place, for example, work harder

Keep feelings to self

Check and double check everything

Try to predict problems before they happen

Keep problems to myself

Say "Yes" to all requests

Concentrate on getting everything correct

Goal

New beliefs
I am OK
I am me
I am free

New rule - It's normal to tell people how I feel

New rule - It's OK to assert my needs

New rule - It's important that I make room for my feelings

New rule - It's OK to make mistakes as long as I learn from them

New behaviours for new rules

Tell others how I feel

Assert myself when I want to do something

Share problems with trusted others

Check things once of just a few times

Validate and accept my feelings

Be myself

Additional worksheets

Old Cycle

Beliefs
I am...............
I am...............
I am...............

Old rule - If am......................
at all times then I will be OK

Old rule - If am......................
at all times then I will be OK

Old rule - If am......................
at all times then I will be OK

Old rule - If am......................
at all times then I will be OK

Old behaviours used to keep rule in place, for example, work harder

_____

_____

_____

_____

_____

_____

Goal

New beliefs
I am...............
I am...............
I am...............

New rule -

New rule -

New rule -

New rule -

New behaviours for new rules

_____

_____

_____

_____

_____

_____

Maintenance cycle based on Christine Padesky's 'Hot Cross Bun' approach

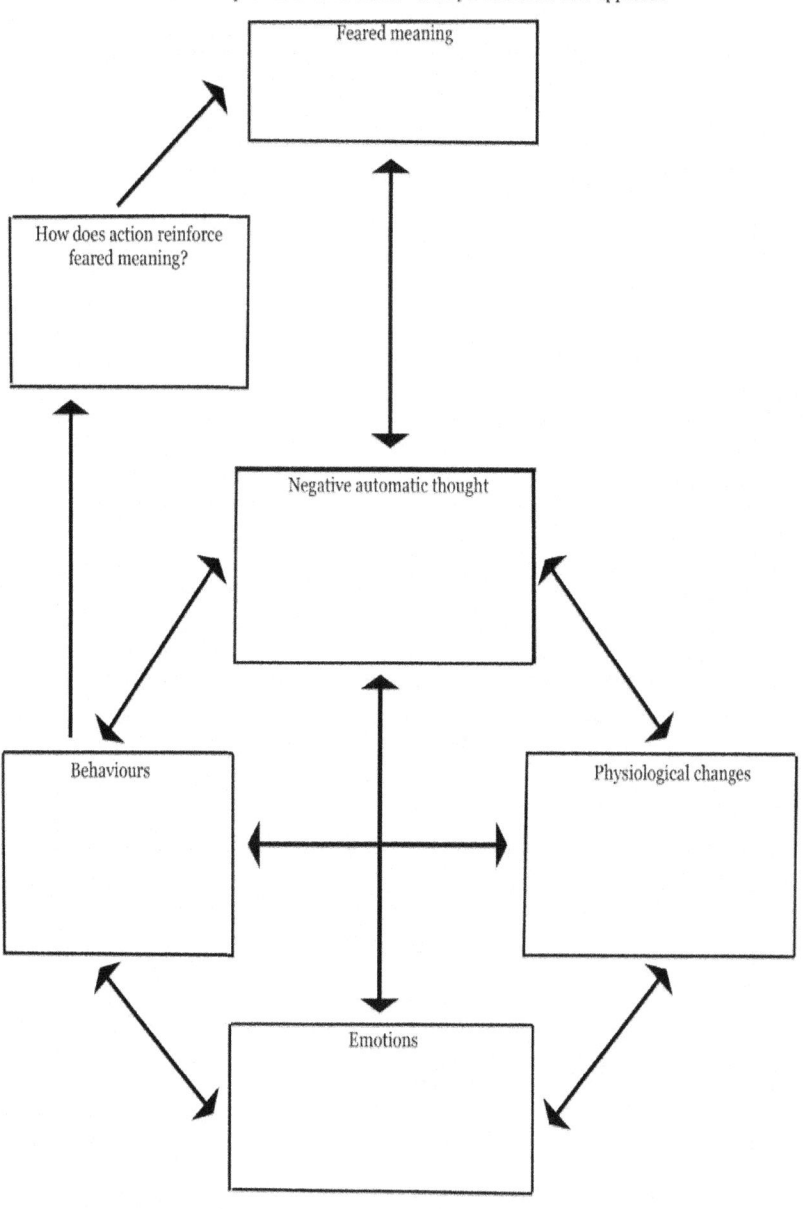

- Feared meaning
- How does action reinforce feared meaning?
- Negative automatic thought
- Behaviours
- Physiological changes
- Emotions

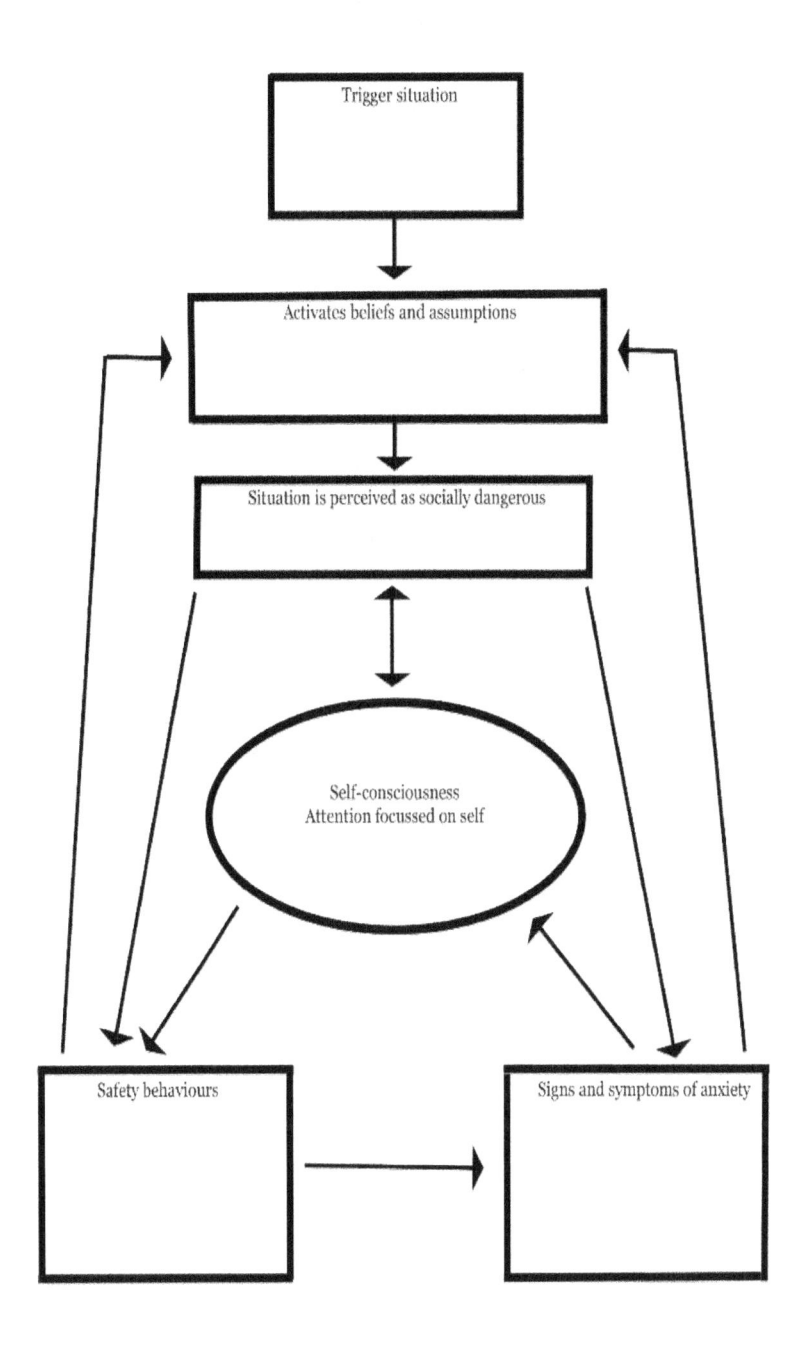

```
                    ┌─────────────────────┐
                    │  Trigger situation  │
                    └──────────┬──────────┘
                               ▼
         ┌──────────────────────────────────────────┐
    ┌───▶│       Activates beliefs and assumptions  │◀───┐
    │    └──────────────────────┬───────────────────┘    │
    │                           ▼                         │
    │    ┌──────────────────────────────────────────┐    │
    │    │  Situation is perceived as socially      │    │
    │    │  dangerous                                │    │
    │    └──────────────────────┬───────────────────┘    │
    │                           ▼                         │
    │                   ┌───────────────┐                 │
    │                   │Self-consciousness│              │
    │                   │Attention focussed│              │
    │                   │   on self        │              │
    │                   └───────────────┘                 │
    │                  ↙               ↘                  │
    │    ┌──────────────────┐   ┌──────────────────────┐ │
    └────│ Safety behaviours│──▶│ Signs and symptoms   │─┘
         │                  │   │ of anxiety           │
         └──────────────────┘   └──────────────────────┘
```

Clarke and Wells maintenance model of anxiety (1995)

Vicious flower model, adapted from Moorey, 2010; Wilson & Veale, 2009

Safety behaviour

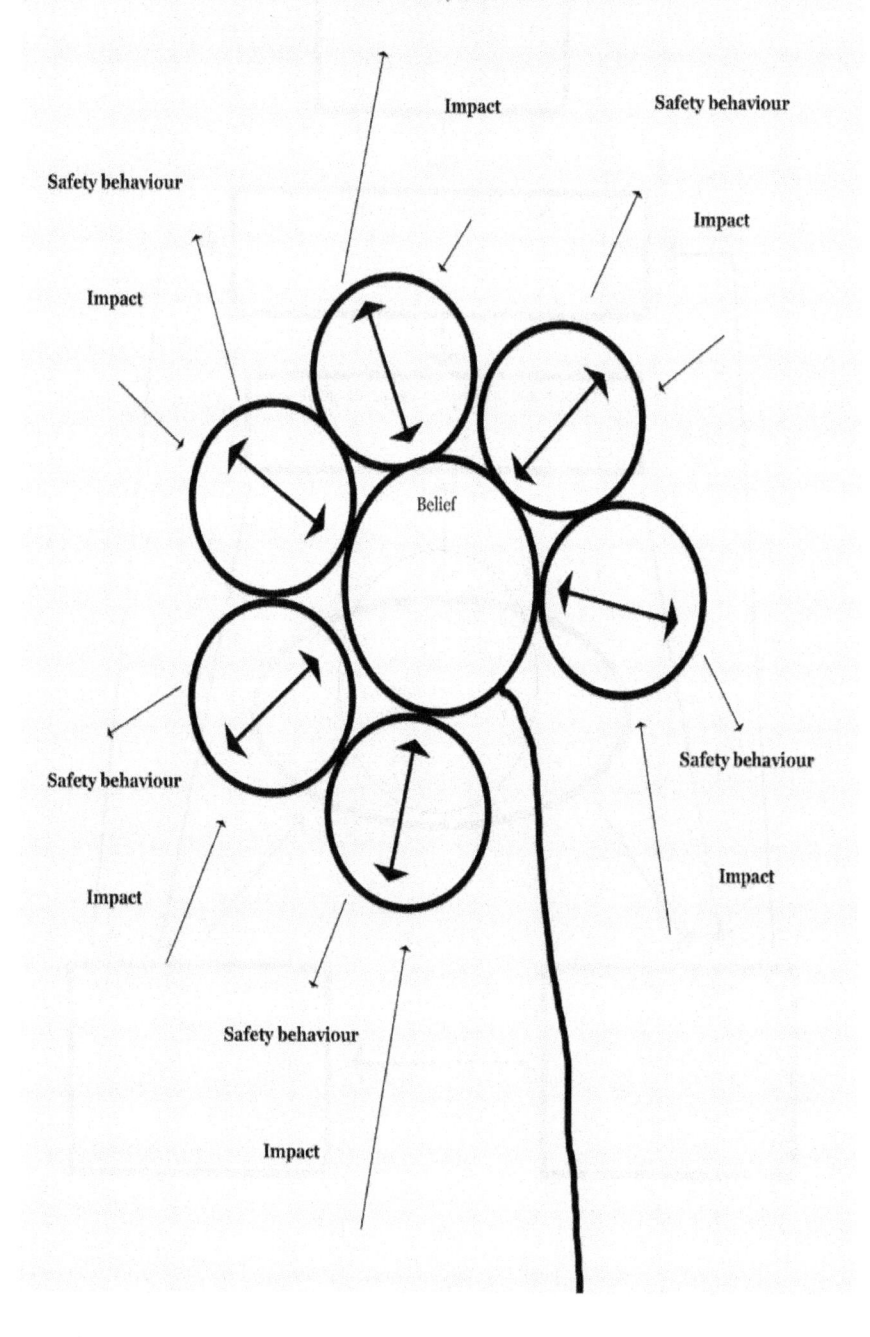

Impact

Safety behaviour

Safety behaviour

Impact

Impact

Belief

Safety behaviour

Safety behaviour

Impact

Impact

Safety behaviour

Impact

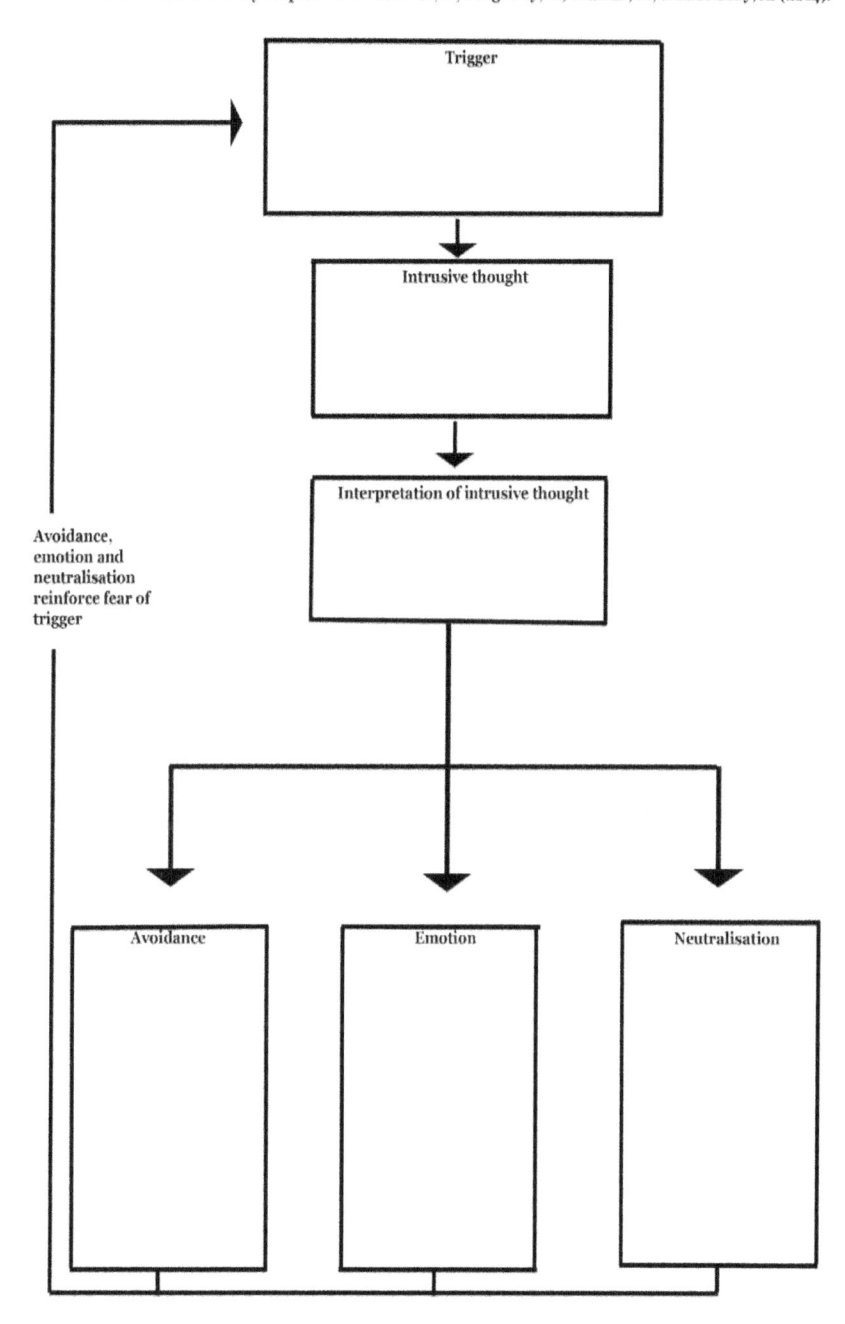

OCD model of anxiety adapted from Rachman, S., Coughtrey, A., Shafran, R., & Radomsky, A. (2014).

```
                    ┌─────────────────┐
          ┌────────▶│     Trigger     │
          │         └────────┬────────┘
          │                  ▼
          │         ┌─────────────────┐
          │         │ Intrusive thought│
          │         └────────┬────────┘
          │                  ▼
          │         ┌──────────────────────────────┐
          │         │ Interpretation of intrusive  │
Avoidance,│         │          thought             │
emotion and         └──────────────┬───────────────┘
neutralisation        ┌────────────┼────────────┐
reinforce fear of     ▼            ▼            ▼
trigger          ┌─────────┐ ┌─────────┐ ┌──────────────┐
          │      │Avoidance│ │ Emotion │ │Neutralisation│
          │      │         │ │         │ │              │
          │      └────┬────┘ └────┬────┘ └──────┬───────┘
          └───────────┴───────────┴─────────────┘
```

Basic OCD cycle

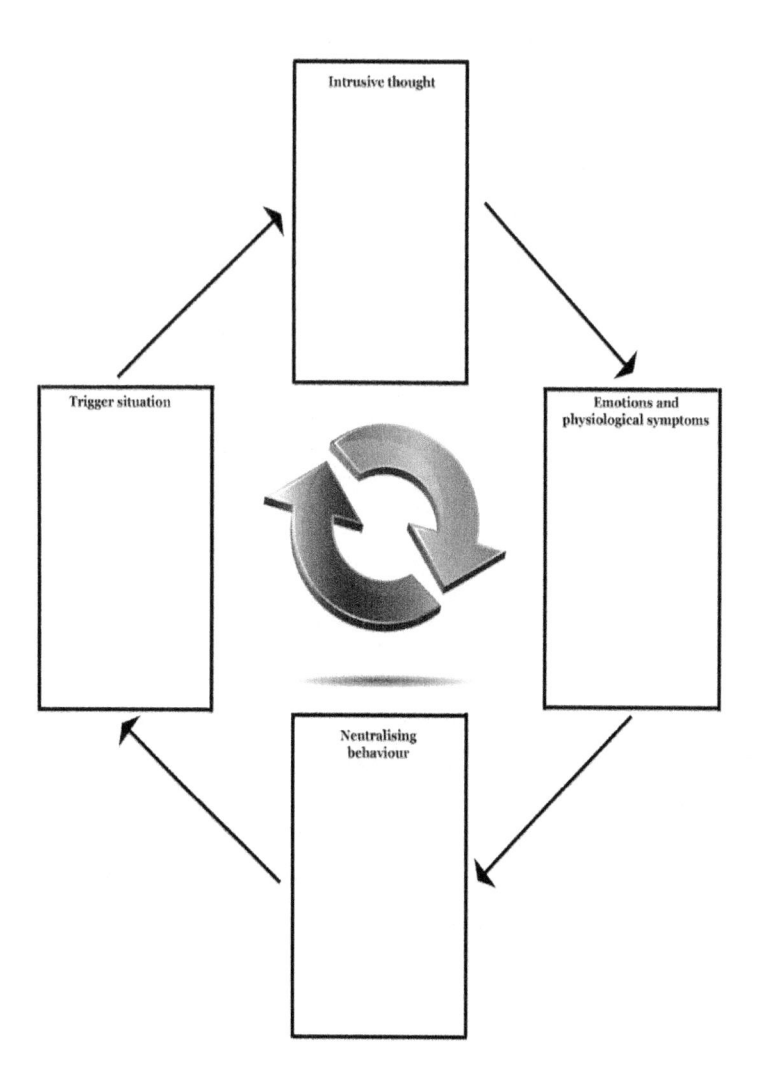

- Intrusive thought
- Trigger situation
- Emotions and physiological symptoms
- Neutralising behaviour

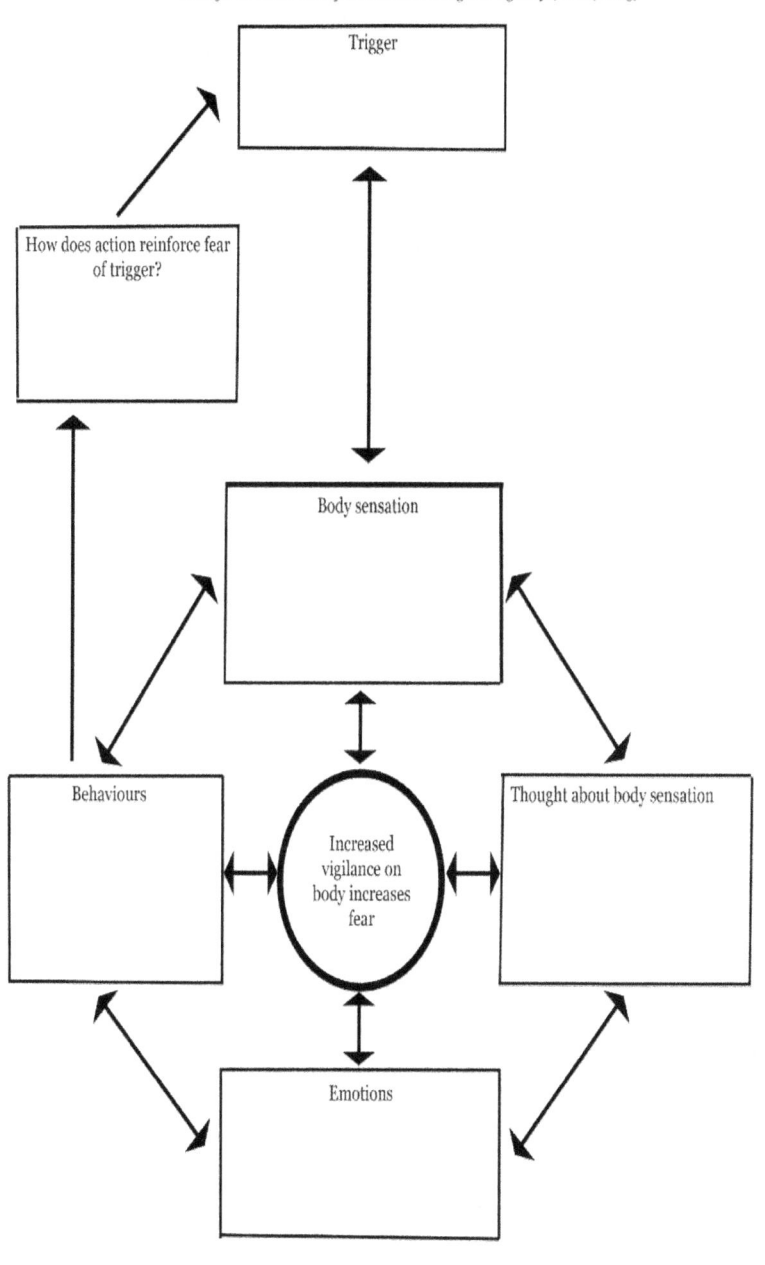

Self-phobic model adapted from Manning & Ridgeway (2008, 2015)

- Trigger
- How does action reinforce fear of trigger?
- Body sensation
- Behaviours
- Thought about body sensation
- Increased vigilance on body increases fear
- Emotions

Maintenance cycle based on Christine Padesky's 'Hot Cross Bun' approach

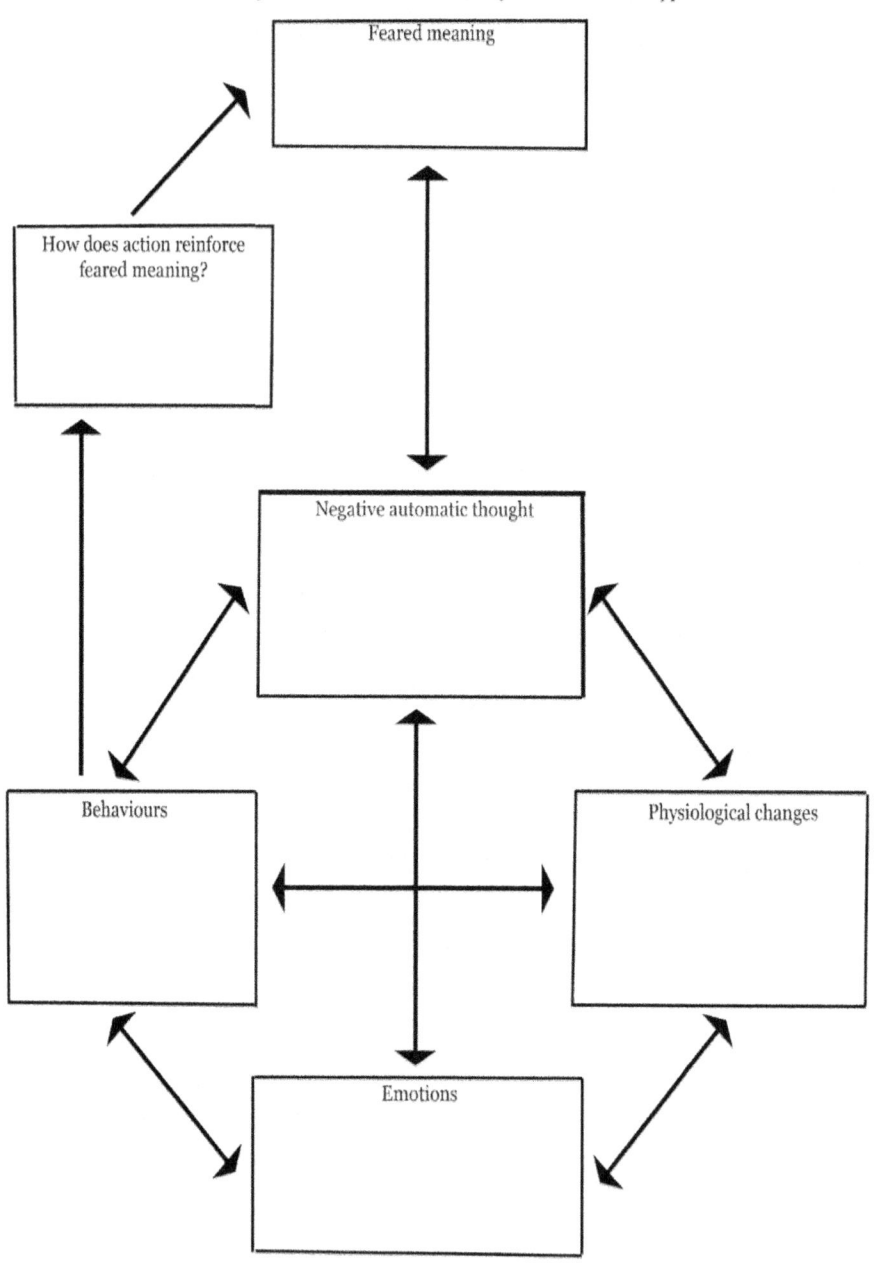

- Feared meaning
- How does action reinforce feared meaning?
- Negative automatic thought
- Behaviours
- Physiological changes
- Emotions

Chapter 13

Making changes using CBT

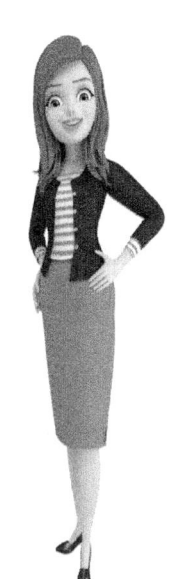

"Luckily there are several different ways that CBT can be used to reduce psychological distress. Psychological problems can be challenged with psychological education, behavioural interventions, cognitive interventions and by using a combined cognitive and behavioural approach. I would like us to define some key concepts for you now so that you become familiar with them when you have your own CBT therapy.

"So Kate can we start with **behavioural strategies**? What are they?"

"A behavioural strategy is making a small adjustment to something that you are doing or by altering your environment in some way. It is usually a good idea to measure what impact behavioural change has on you. For example, let's imagine that there is a lady with health anxiety. When she starts feeling anxious about her health, she might screen her body for symptoms and then go onto the internet to research what might be wrong with her. When she does this she accesses more frightening information, becomes even more anxious and ends up making repeated appointments with her doctor."

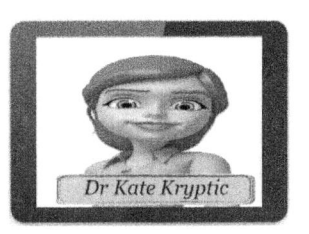

"A new strategy that she might work on with her therapist is to use postponement. She learns to postpone screening her body and put off going onto the internet. When she does this she finds that her anxiety starts to reduce and it becomes easier to stop screening her body and going onto the internet. She then starts to feel less anxious about her health and makes less appointments with her doctor. If she finds the new strategy works for her she can learn from it and repeat it again in the future."

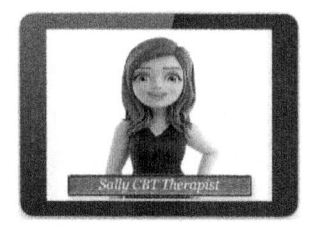

"Thanks for that Kate. Now can you tell our readers about **cognitive interventions**?"

"Cognitive interventions are strategies that you can use mainly within your mind. In particular, cognitive interventions may require you to challenge the contents of your thoughts to improve the way that you feel. Cognitive strategies, which we will cover a bit more later on, may also involve telling yourself something along the lines of "It's just a thought" when you have frightening thoughts or challenging the accuracy of frightening thoughts. These types of exercises tend to work more successfully when distress levels are lower. This is because, as we discussed earlier, the neocortex which is used more so for cognitive approaches tends to go off-line or has reduced capacity at times of heightened distress."

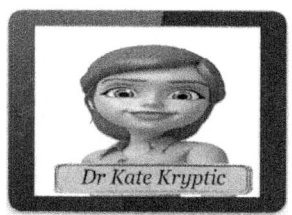

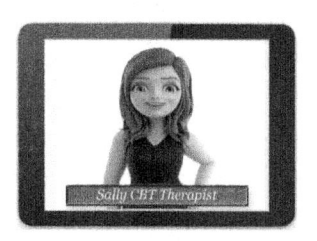

"And cognitive behaviour therapy?"

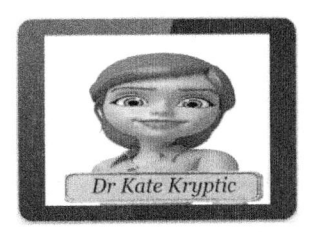

"To make long-lasting changes to their symptoms of distress our readers will eventually need to use a combined **cognitive and behavioural approach**. This will involve using cognitive and behavioural tools, at the same time, while challenging previously feared thoughts and behaviours."

"One thing I really like about CBT is that its models explain in a straightforward, scientific way how people's emotional problems occur. Arguably, more importantly, CBT also highlights factors that continue to maintain people's problems and explains what people can do to reduce their emotional distress and suffering."

Chapter 14

Challenging negative automatic thoughts

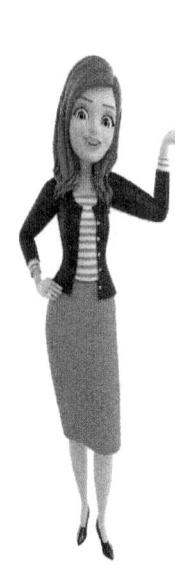

"A practice that many cognitive behaviour therapists teach is recognition of **negative automatic thoughts** or **NATS** for short. Can you tell us why this is the case Kate?"

"OK. The first thing that I'd like to share with our readers is that NATS are the types of thought that run in the back of our mind when we complete many day to day activities. NATS are likely to be in operation for many individuals who are depressed or anxious. NATs are important to identify because they affect the way that we feel."

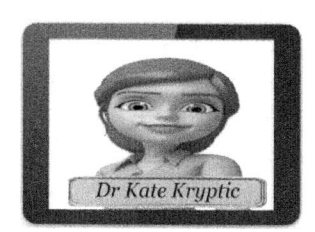

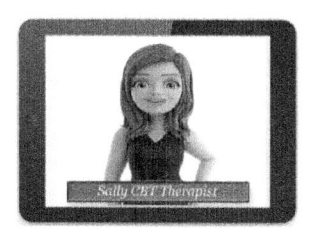

"Kate how do you help your clients recognise their NATS?"

"The first stage in recognising NATS is to set aside some time before or after events that provoke more intense emotion and write down the types of automatic thoughts that come to mind."

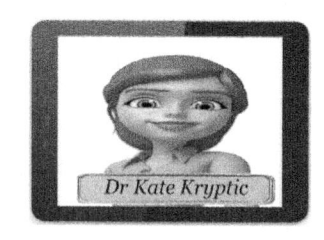

152

"On the following page I have placed a list of common thoughts experienced by individuals with **social anxiety**. Social anxiety is a type of anxiety, where people become anxious before, during or after interactions with others. People with social anxiety often attempt to hide their anxiety, or attempt to avoid social situations where they might become anxious."

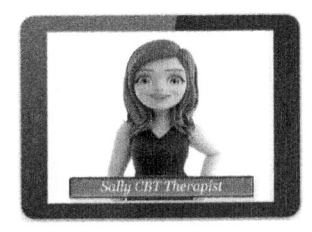

"Have you chosen social anxiety as an example because people with social anxiety have more NATS than people with other types of mental health problems?"

"No, I could easily have picked health anxiety, depression, or many other different types of mental health issues. NATS are common to all conditions."

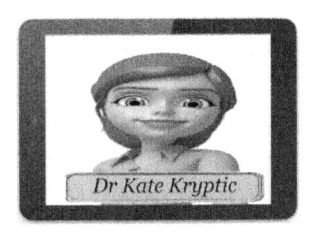

Common automatic thoughts in social anxiety

"People will find me boring"
"My shaking will give me away"
"People aren't interested in finding out what I have to say"
"People won't mind if I leave early"
"I look odd"
"I have nothing to contribute"
"People don't invite me anywhere"
"I look stupid"
"I have no social skills"
"They won't mind if I cancel, in fact they will be relieved"
"I am boring ... Everyone is looking at me"
"I am making a fool of myself"
"I'm not coming across very well"

"They can see how nervous I am"
"I am going to say something stupid"
"She doesn't like you, it's obvious!"
"He's trying to humiliate you"
"My face looks like a tomato. I look ugly"
"They think that I'm inept"
"They don't really want me to come

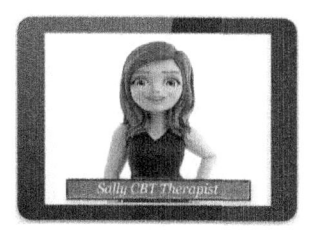

"So if our readers notice their NATS what do they do next?"

"Once our readers recognise that they have NATS they then have a choice about how they decide to react to them. They can either challenge them, or become aware of them, and choose not to react to them. Many of my clients find that noticing their negative thoughts, and choosing not to react to them is very difficult, initially. With this in mind, I often find it useful in the early stages to spend more time challenging NATS with my clients."

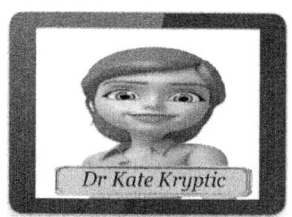

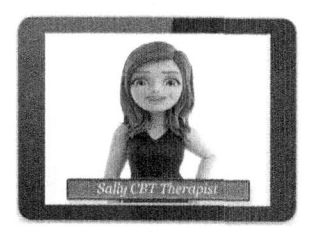

"What do you think is the best way to challenge NATS?"

"One of the most effective ways to challenge NATS is to bring alternative explanations to mind. I have placed a section of a

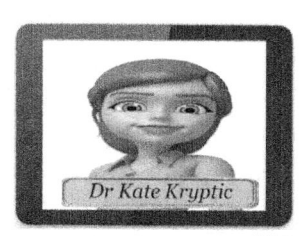

thought challenging record on the next page from one of my clients with social anxiety. A thought challenging record is really a collection of notes that our readers can make to provide alternative evidence against their NATS. Our readers can find empty tables at the back of this chapter that they can photocopy and use to challenge their NATS. Larger CBT sheets can be found in our other book CBT worksheets. Negative automatic thoughts are placed in the first column, evidence for the NATS are placed in the second column, evidence against the NAT is placed in the third column, and an alternative more balanced thoughts is placed in the fourth column."

NAT challenging form

Negative automatic thought, for example, "I will be a laughing stock!"	Evidence for negative automatic thought, for example, "I feel that it might happen"	Evidence against negative automatic thought, for example, this has never happened before	New more balanced thought, for example, although I feel anxious nothing has happend in the past and is unlikely to happen this time
I will be a laughing stock when I eat with Laura's family	I feel that people will judge me. I behave oddly Sometimes people feel awkward around me	No one has laughed at me for a long time. Laura's family like me. Laura still wants to be in a relationship with me. No one has said anything. Most people don't notice anxiety or they don't really care	I feel anxious, but no one seems to notice or they don't care.

To help my clients understand the power of NATS I often place their NATS into a Padesky cycle. I have placed one of Ben's NATs into a Padesky cycle below. This makes it a bit more obvious about the impact that NAT's can have and is a very good starting point to challenge them."

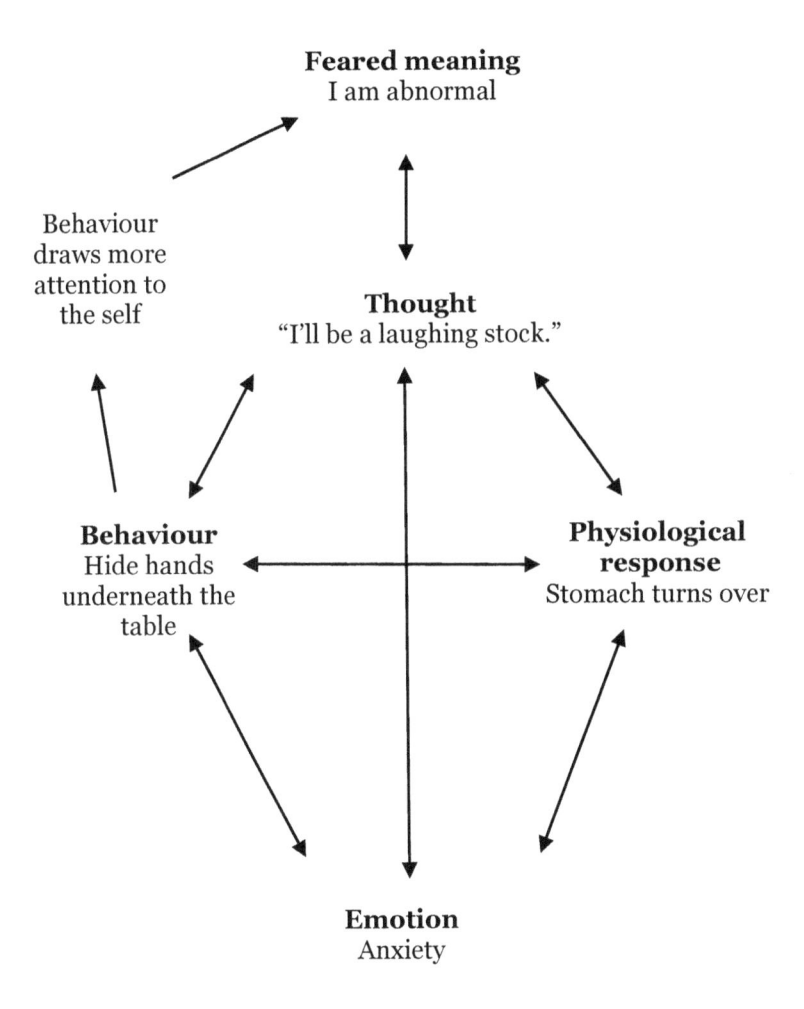

Feared meaning
I am abnormal

Behaviour draws more attention to the self

Thought
"I'll be a laughing stock."

Behaviour
Hide hands underneath the table

Physiological response
Stomach turns over

Emotion
Anxiety

"Collecting evidence against NATS can sometimes be difficult and because of this it will be important to persist. Some people find it helpful to complete NAT challenging exercises with their therapist. Alternatively, our readers might ask trusted loved ones to help them challenge their NATS, or our readers could think about what they might say to others with similar problems to themselves when challenging their NATS."

"After completing a thought challenging record it is often useful to put the alternative more balanced thought into another Padesky cycle and look at how it might change things. I have placed Ben's example below."

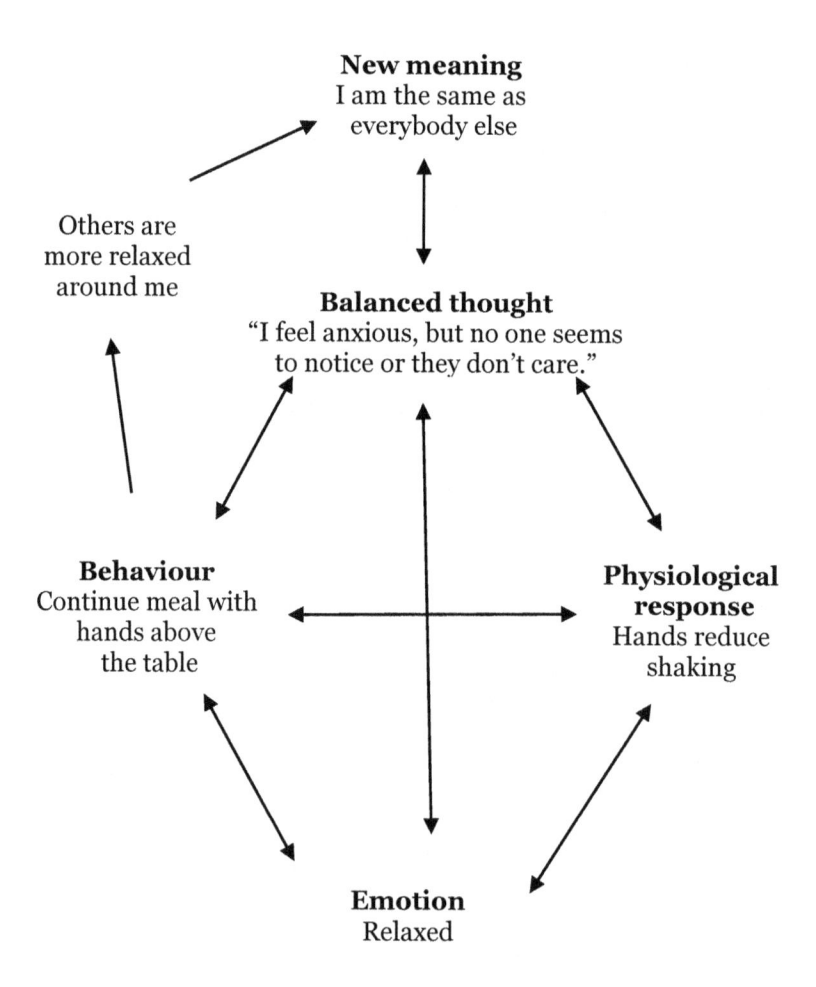

New meaning
I am the same as everybody else

Others are more relaxed around me

Balanced thought
"I feel anxious, but no one seems to notice or they don't care."

Behaviour
Continue meal with hands above the table

Physiological response
Hands reduce shaking

Emotion
Relaxed

"NATS often have a habit of coming back, so it may be useful for our readers get their NAT challenging notes out and re-read them when this occurs. In her book "Overcoming Social Anxiety and Shyness" Professor Gillian Butler recommends the use of flash cards. She suggests that people make cards with their NAT's on one side and place alternative more balanced thoughts on the other. Taking a small card out from time to time in various situations can then be used as a memory aid. Knowing the card is there without needing to look at it can also jog the memory. I have placed some blank thoughts challenging sheets and Padesky positive cycles for our clients to complete if they want to."

NAT challenging form

Negative automatic thought, for example, "I will be a laughing stock!"	Evidence for negative automatic thought, for example, "I feel that it might happen"	Evidence against negative automatic thought, for example, this has never happened before	New more balanced thought, for example, although I feel anxious nothing has happend in the past and is unlikely to happen this time

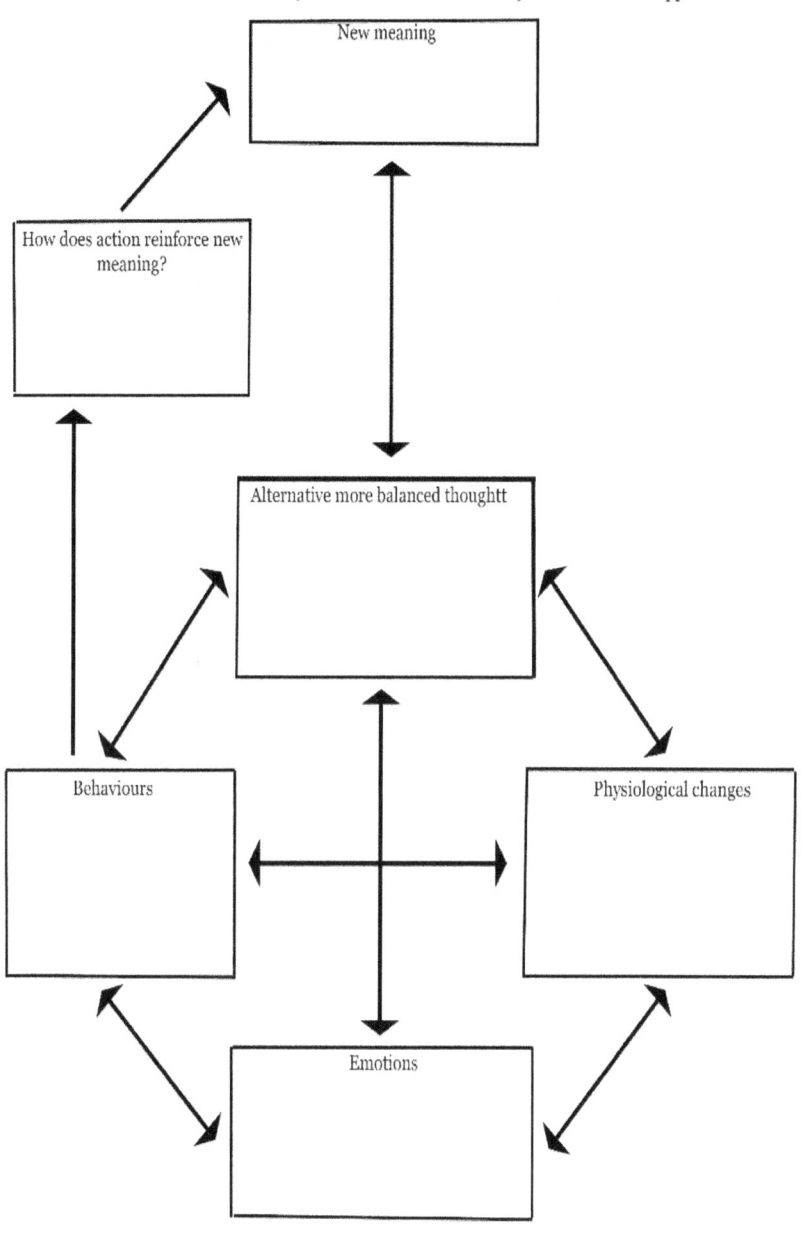

Positive maintenance cycle based on Christine Padesky's 'Hot Cross Bun' approach

- New meaning
- How does action reinforce new meaning?
- Alternative more balanced thoughtt
- Behaviours
- Physiological changes
- Emotions

Chapter 15

Working with emotions

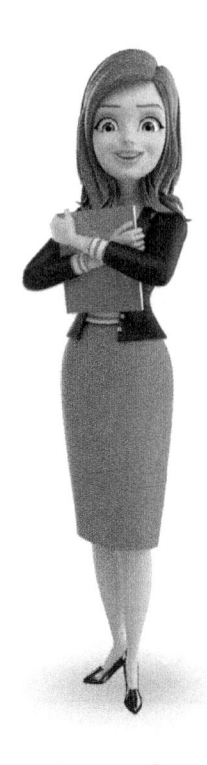

"Most CBT therapists will spend a good deal of their therapy time helping clients to recognise their feelings and to form an improved relationship with their emotions. Often, feelings such as anxiety, anger, guilt, low mood, and shame are viewed as a threat, or are seen as bodily experiences that need to be feared or hidden. As a result, many clients use strategies such as ignoring feelings, controlling feelings, distracting the self from feelings, hiding feelings, and using safety behaviours. This results in their distress being kept at quite a high level. What do you do to help people understand this Kate?"

"I once worked with a young teacher called Jemma. She sat in front of me, shifting around continuously in her chair, rubbing the back of her neck, breathing from the top of her chest, sighing and holding her breath at various times. She appeared to be a real thinker and was able to talk about her difficulties quite easily. She was telling me how problems arose between herself and one of her friends, and she had understood her part in the falling out. When I asked Jemma how she was feeling in her body she found it extremely difficult to answer. It wasn't the case that Jemma didn't experience emotions as she was displaying them quite evidently in front of me, through her body language. It was more simply a case that

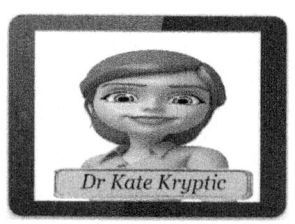

Jemma felt very uncomfortable when she recognised her bodily sensations of anxiety and felt a lot better when she remained in her head. When I asked Jemma if she had ever developed any good ways to soothe her anxiety she couldn't think of any. She stated quite simply that she was brought up as a child in a home where people didn't talk about their feelings. As a result of this from a very early age Jemma had naturally developed many sophisticated ways of ignoring or controlling her emotions and in fact had become quite an expert in ignoring her feelings."

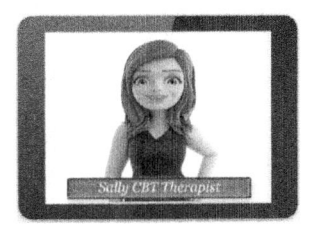

"How can you help somebody who doesn't feel their emotions? I thought CBT only works if people understand how they are feeling!"

"Well you're right in that we really do need to help our clients notice they are having feelings for CBT to work effectively. Where we can start is by gently encouraging our clients to begin observing what is happening in their body more, and then building a relationship with their feelings."

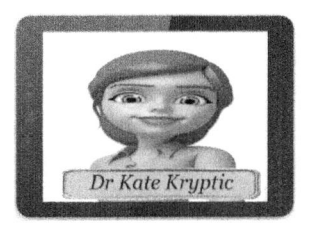

"I have drawn a diagram on the next page which shows how many people react to their emotions, in this case I have used anxiety as an example."

Anxiety worked example

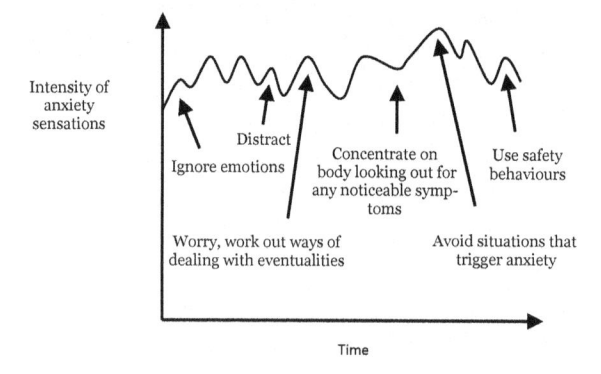

[Figure: Graph showing intensity of anxiety sensations over time, with peaks labelled: Distract, Concentrate on body looking out for any noticeable symptoms, Use safety behaviours; and troughs labelled: Ignore emotions, Worry, work out ways of dealing with eventualities, Avoid situations that trigger anxiety.]

"This drawing demonstrates the relationship between our natural attempts to control or avoid anxiety and our overall level of anxiety sensations."

"In my sessions I ask my clients - What would happen if you tried the opposite of the above? For example, instead of ignoring emotions, you notice them and tell them that it is fine for them to be there.

What if instead of distracting yourself from anxiety, you focus on your anxiety and spend time in your body rather than in your head.

I also ask what would happen if you begin to see anxiety as a friend rather than your enemy, if you allow your anxiety to be visible rather than try to hide it, and give permission for your anxiety to stay, rather than trying to get rid of it as soon as possible?

I often draw a table out on my whiteboard. I have placed a copy of it on the next page."

Commonly applied natural solutions to anxiety	Strategy based on an opposite approach
Avoid uncomfortable feelings	Approach uncomfortable feelings
Distract self – Keep mind off of feelings	Focus on feelings
Perceive anxiety symptoms as threatening. Try to hide symptoms	Perceive anxiety as part of the body that works for us. Embrace symptoms and allow symptoms to be visible
Control anxiety, try to extinguish symptoms as soon as possible	Allow anxiety to stay for as long as it wants
Tell emotions that they shouldn't be there	Tell emotions that there are good reasons for them being there

"The ideas covered in the right hand column of the above table often confuses my clients, because it feels so alien to them. Maybe not dissimilar to someone asking them to grab a red-hot poker, while this person assures them that it is not going to harm them. This type of **'counter-intuitive'** strategy to anxiety is the last thing that most people who experience emotional distress would want to do as they feel that their distress will rise significantly. By the way, when I say counter-intuitive I mean people carrying out behaviours or engaging in thoughts which are the direct opposite of what people's intuition or feelings tell them is right."

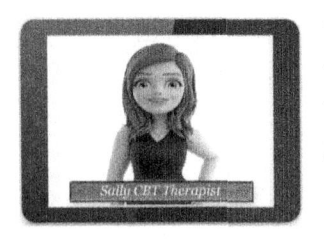

"So how do you help people to do this exercise, especially if they think their painful feelings might get even worse?"

"I start by returning to the ideas that we discussed in the early chapters of this book. We have the neo-cortex at the top of the brain, the prefrontal cortex underneath that, and the sub-cortical regions at the bottom of the brain. A slight problem with people who become highly distressed or anxious is that their pre-frontal cortex tends to go off-line at this point. In this respect, they could find themselves in situations, when they are upset, with their minds going blank, and finding it very difficult to think clearly or rationally."

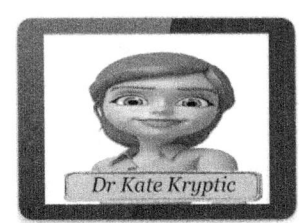

"With this in mind, I suggest to my clients that a very useful starting point is to begin viewing themselves as a bit like a parent to the subcortical or primitive regions of the brain. I ask clients to imagine this part of the brain not as the enemy but more like a servant that has worked for them loyally and tirelessly in the background, but who is also very rarely appreciated for his or her effort."

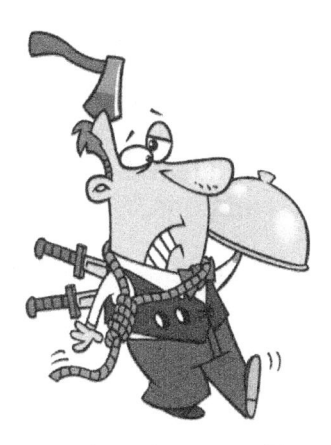

"I've got a niggling feeling that somethings not quite right"

"I suggest that they begin to use their new parenting approach when they are on their own and when their distressing emotions are mild. Mild distress may be around, when our readers have day to day problems, for example, a problem at work, a problem with a friend or a relative etc. Mild distress may also be around when they worry, or when they ask "What if?" questions. The essence of the approach that I am going to suggest our readers use, is to become more aware of their feelings, especially painful feelings at the earliest stage possible."

"The best way to explain is with a demonstration. Would you mind helping me with this Jemma?"

"Yes! Sure!"

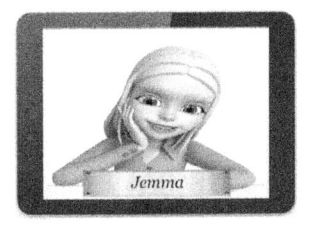

Jemma

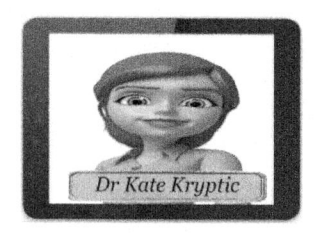

"OK Jemma I would just like you to think of a problem that you have had just recently, a problem that when you think about it now, still leaves you feeling slightly anxious."

"OK, I've thought of something. Do you want me to talk to you about it?"

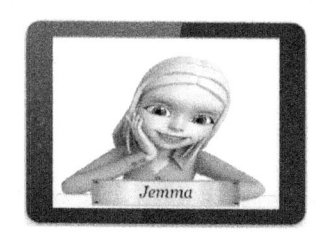

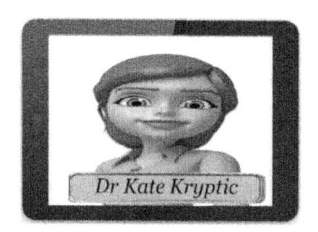

"No I'd like you to keep it to yourself for now. I'd just like you to think about where you feel your emotion more strongly."

"I feel it most in my chest!"

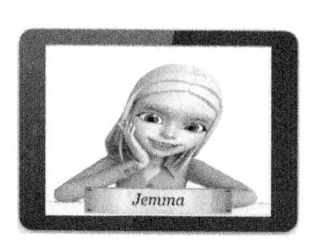

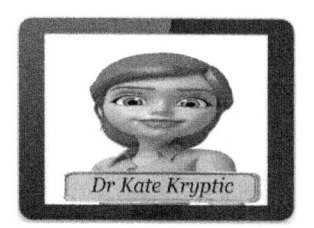

"Good. Keep your focus there. Now place one of your hands on your chest in the place where you feel your emotion more strongly. You are placing your hand on your body where your emotion is, because many of us who are prone to avoiding emotions unconsciously and automatically move away from feeling emotions, and go into our heads instead. You are

168

gaining a connection with your emotions and keeping your focus on how you are feeling."

"Placing your hand on the part of your body where you feel your anxiety more strongly will also act as a reminder to you, to keep your focus on your emotions. It is very important while you are doing this exercise to focus on feeling your feelings and remind yourself that you really are willing for your emotions to be there."

"Focussing on the part of your body underneath you hand with your mind, examine exactly what your emotion feels like. For example, how much space do your feelings take up? How painful or uncomfortable are your feelings. Jemma, can you rate the intensity of your feeling between 1 and 10, where 10 is the highest level of intensity?"

"They're about a 7 at the moment."

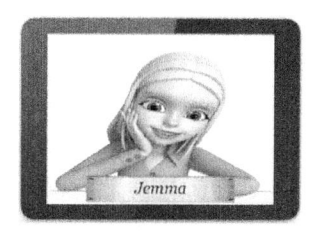

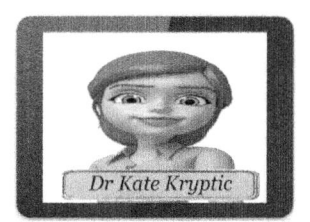

"OK, while you continue to feel your anxiety, mentally give it your permission to take up the space that it is taking up in your body. Taking things a little further I would also like you to speak internally with your anxiety saying something along the lines of the following."

"Thank you for being there" … "There are very good reasons for you being there."

"Keep in mind the idea that from the primitive minds point of view there is a good reason for your anxiety being there, even if it does not make sense logically."

"Now follow that by saying "You are welcome to stay there for as long as you want."

"Bear in mind again Jemma from the primitive mind's point of view that if it notices during its screening process that there is a cue to a potential threat, which may be physical or psychological, it is just doing its job properly if it brings the threat to your attention and helps you to prepare. The threat does not need to be logical, real or valid in the current time mode. If it has been perceived as a threat in the past, or you have previously confirmed the existence of the threat by withdrawing from this threat in the past, then from the primitive mind's point of view the threat is still active."

"While feeling your symptoms of anxiety it is important when you speak to your feelings that you really mean what you are saying. Let go of all your thoughts and focus on your feeling. The importance of your self-communication is not in the words that you use but rather your intention behind your words. Keep an idea in mind of accepting, recognising, being grateful and being patient. I'm just going to ask you to do this for a minute Kate and we will see what happens."

...a minute passes...

"What are you noticing at the moment Jemma?"

"The feeling is going down...It's about a 4 now."

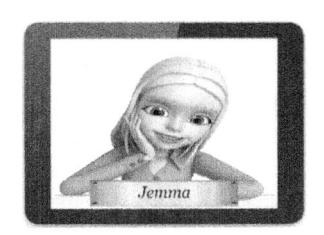

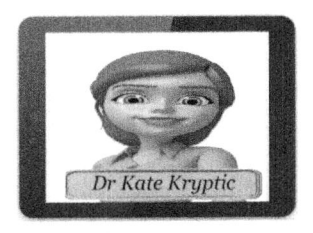

"OK staying with the feeling, noticing that it is going down. Just stay with it. We'll see what happens in another minute or so."

...another minute passes...

"OK, Jemma what are you noticing now?"

"It's gone!"

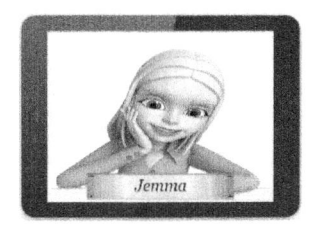

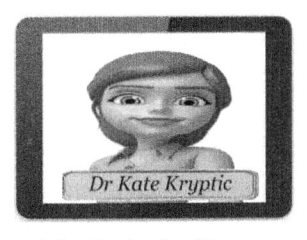

"Thanks for helping our readers with that Jemma. It is important in the early stages of CBT that when our readers are experiencing anxiety, low mood, guilt and anger to practice being with their feelings as much as possible. This will help them in two ways. Firstly, it will help them to fear their feelings less and secondly it will make it more likely that they will be able to use this acceptance approach when they are experiencing higher levels of distress. Our readers will need to bear in mind that in a state of heightened distress the frontal lobes where most of our logical thinking occurs stop working somewhat. Doing the same thing over and over again when they are not so distressed will make it more likely that they will be able to access and use this approach automatically when they really need it."

"Professor Knutt. Do you have anything you can add here in terms of scientific processes?

"Yes. If you can cast your mind back to when we talked about the basal ganglia earlier. When we become highly distressed we are likely to continue to return to our old unhelpful habitual behaviours due to the strong influence of sub-cortical regions of our brains. As I mentioned earlier when we become highly anxious, the sub-cortical region of the brain becomes dominant and this part of the brain encourages the use of repetitive habits. This can lead us to do the same things that we have always done before."

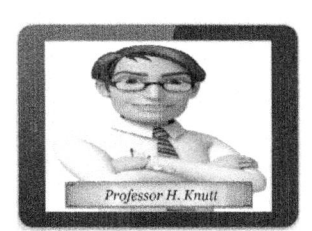

"To change the use of unhelpful habits, our readers will need to practice using the new exercises that they will learn in their therapy over and over again. Eventually, these new habits will come into place automatically when our readers are faced with distressing situations. This process takes time, however, as brain wiring does not grow instantaneously."

Chapter 16

Breaking patterns of worry and rumination

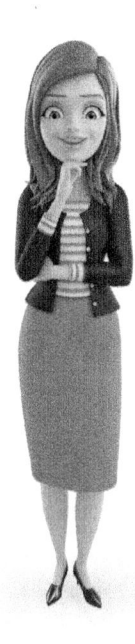

"Most people who experience mental health problems will spend a significant portion of their time ruminating or worrying. Because these processes tend to maintain emotional difficulties it is not uncommon for them to be discussed in CBT sessions."

"We'll talk about **rumination** first. Rumination is a process of churning negative thoughts over in one's mind. Most ruminative thoughts are connected to the self and the past. Some people suggest that rumination is helpful because it can help to create lots of possibilities, and can offer solutions when we are faced with specific problems. Rumination, however, does not work well when we try to analyse our way out of low-mood."

"Kate would you be able to tell us how people fall into patterns of rumination?"

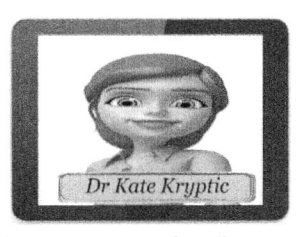

"A process of rumination is kept in place by the questions we ask ourselves. For example, if we ask "Why does this keep happening to me" or "What's wrong with me?" The questions that we ask ourselves throw up answers which, in turn, can lead us to ask more questions. Before long, if this process continues unstopped we can end up confirming our worst fears, for example, that we are worthless, wrong, useless, bad and such like. The irony of the whole process is that in our search for ways to avoid current or future painful feelings by ruminating, we end up dwelling on the past and we can end up feeling worse than ever. It's not dissimilar to using a shovel to dig ourselves out of a hole. The more we dig, the deeper the hole gets! The problem is that often we do not feel that we have any other way of solving our problems, so we continue to use the same strategy, even though we know it does not work."

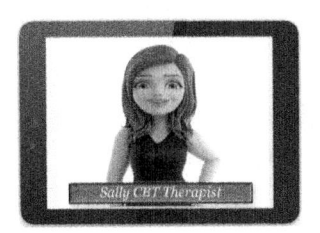

Sally CBT Therapist

"So Kate how is worry similar or different to ruminating?"

Worry is similar to ruminating in that it is also a process of thought churning. The main difference is that worry is focussed on the future and being able to cope with potential outcomes."

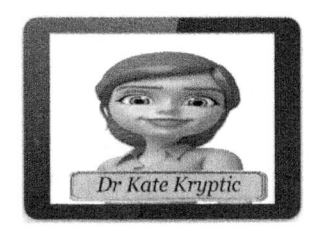

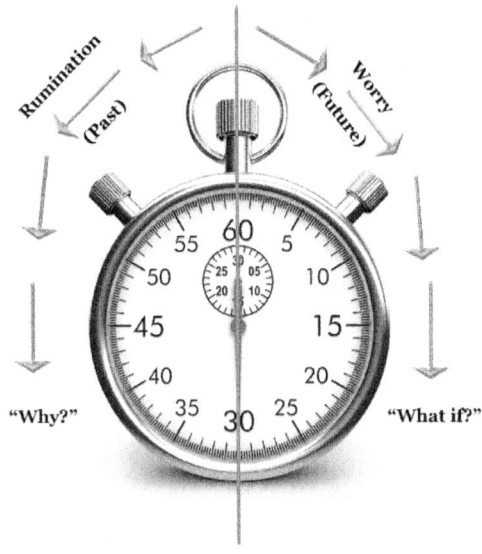

Dr Kate Kryptic

Rumination (Past) — "Why?"

Worry (Future) — "What if?"

"When people worry they think about upcoming situations and ask questions such as "What will I do if this happens?" "What is the worst thing that could happen?" or "What if this happens?" They do this because they think that if they can imagine the worst case scenario, then they will be able to put things in place to deal with whatever happens in a particular situation. They think if they can work out what might happen in advance then they will be safe. Ironically, however, just like rumination, in an attempt to achieve certainty and to feel safe, we can end up feeling more frightened than ever, and also experience frightening intrusive thoughts."

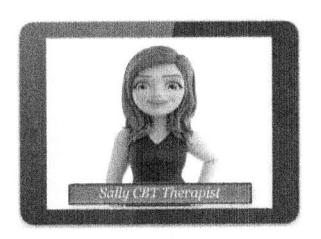

"Intrusive thoughts?"

"An intrusive thought is a thought that pushes its way into awareness with extreme urgency. Intrusive thoughts often appear to come out of nowhere and carry high levels of emotional distress with them. Ironically, intrusive thoughts alone can trigger heightened anxiety."

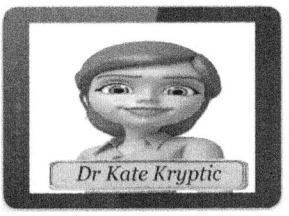

"Before I explain why intrusive thoughts may occur, I want to offer a simple analogy about the functioning of the mind for our readers."

"First I'd like our readers to recognise that they have a **conscious mind.** When people use their conscious minds they are awake to thoughts, images or sensations that they experience. I'd like us to imagine that the conscious mind is a bit like a magic white board that begins to erase what is written on it after only a few seconds. Because the ink or information expressed using the ink disappears so rapidly the only way to keep anything live on this white board is to continuously write on it over and over again. When new information is written on the white board, information that was on the white board previously, disappears even more rapidly. A further point to note is that the amount of information that can be written on the whiteboard at any one point in time is limited due to the whiteboards small size."

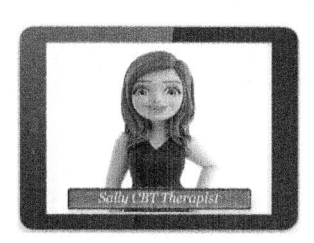

"So Kate are you saying the mind is like a whitebead. I'm not sure I understand?

"Do you mind if I demonstrate with you Sally? It's much easier to show our readers how this works rather than to explain it. Before we start I just want to let you know that this is not a test. It's just a little exercise so that you can find out how much information your mind can hold onto. I am going to start by asking you to remember five randon numbers and letters. Are you ready?

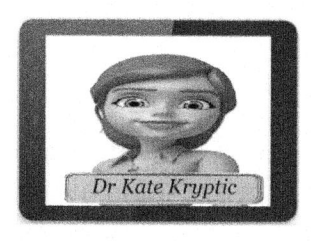

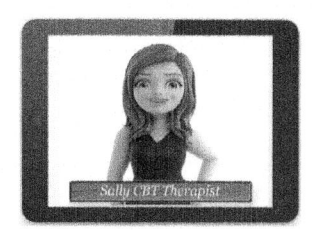

"Yes"

176

"5A3KQ. Have you got that?"

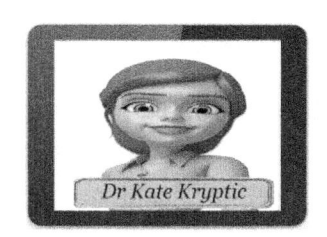

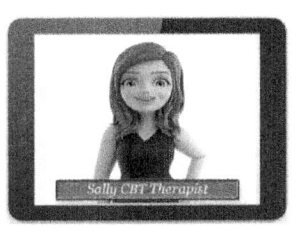

"Yes. I think so!"

"Alright I now want you to remember these numbers as well."

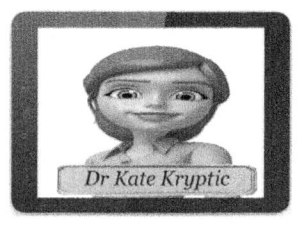

"27KR1..."Right Sally, can you repeat that sequence for me?"

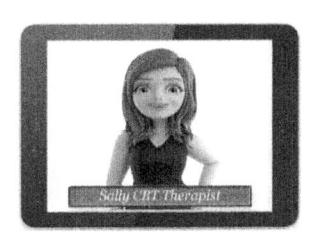

"27KR1"

"Good...And, the first sequence"

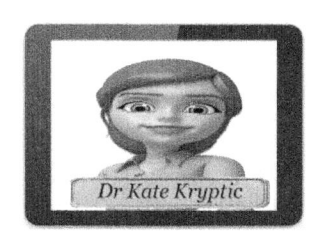

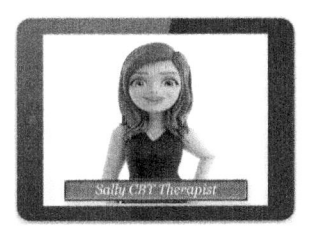

"...Erm...[a big pause follows] ...57...Q...It seems to have gone out of my head... I'm sorry."

177

"There's no need to be sorry Sally. This is exactly what is meant to happen. This is how the mind works. We just gave your internal whiteboard an impossible task. Hardly anyone can recall over 9 randomly presented units of information unless they use specialised memory techniques, and I just gave you 10. That's why I'm saying the whiteboard is small in size."
"I'll just explain it a bit more. A benefit of the white board's disappearing ink process is that it is constantly available for continuous use. As a result of this, huge amounts of information can be written on the whiteboard during the period of its lifetime. In many respects, it could be suggested that we could feel grateful that the whiteboard loses access to information so quickly. If it didn't it would quite quickly become jammed up with too much information and become unusable."

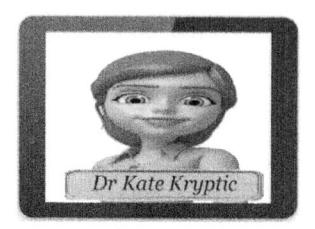

"Taking this idea further, I'd like us to imagine that our **out of conscious processes** work a little bit like a building that the white board is housed in. For our readers benefit I'll just explain that out of conscious processes are brain functions that we are unaware of, or mental processes that go on in the back of our minds."

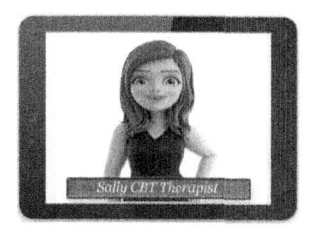

"And, what's the significance of associating the out of conscious mind with a building?"

"I'm saying that out of conscious processes are like a building because the amount of brain space required for out of conscious thinking is absolutely huge in in comparison to the amount of brain used for the white board. The building is also three dimensional unlike the two dimensional whiteboard, there are also multiple rooms, and secret passageways.

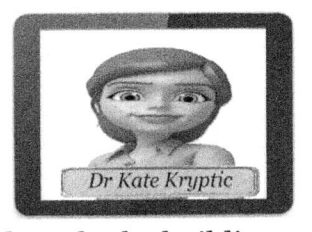

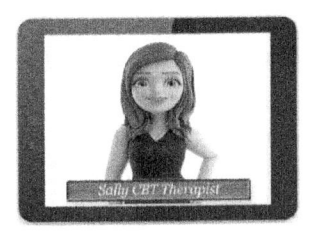

"I understand why it is big but what does the three dimensional layout of the building represent, with multiple rooms and such like?"

"This represents an idea that the out of conscious mind can think on several different levels at the same time. It can absorb information from our environment, take care of all of our bodily functions, plan our activities, assist our communication, and think about problems we have in our lives without us being aware of it. It can also use symbols, images, and words to create ideas and connect them up in a way that we would struggle to do consciously. What it can do is really quite incredible!"

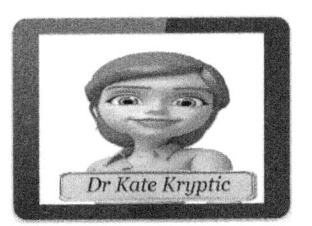

"In this building there are also filing cabinets crammed with information that we thought we had forgotten about, and there are reams of papers lying around waiting to be filed."

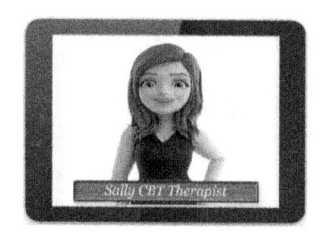

"What do the reams of papers represent?"

"The reams of paper represent thoughts that we have not fully processed or ideas that we are currently working on. Many people may have several hundred or even thousands of different thoughts strands they are working on at any one time. Thought strands may be about relationships with different people, hobbies or interests, work projects, holidays and such like. Information does not disappear easily from this building but very often it can get lost or misfiled."

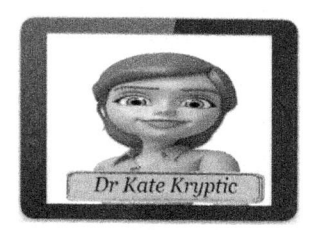

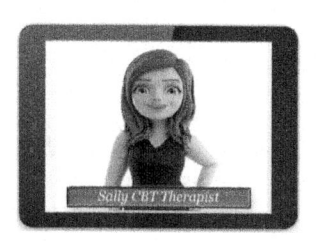

"So how does it get lost or misfiled?"

"There is so much information in this building or in peoples' minds that sometimes it is hard for them to find what they are looking for. The more information that's in the building the harder it is to find what they need."

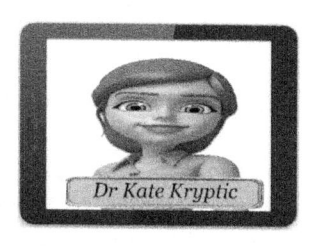

"Now imagine that in this building there is a little librarian who is very loyal to you and will try to find answers to anything that you ask using the whiteboard, even if it means working through the night. Sometimes the librarian finds information quickly, sometimes it might take days, but when the librarian finds answers to questions posed on the whiteboard it will post it an answer on the whiteboard just as soon as space becomes available."

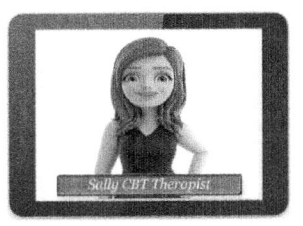

"I'm still not sure I still fully understand this analogy of a librarian Kate. How does this work with real problems?"

"OK. Let's imagine that Jemma is walking down the street one day and on the other side of the street there is a girl whose face she recognises. She is immediately aware that she knows her but this is not where she usually sees her. She asks herself "Where do I know her from?" a few times. Nothing comes to her mind immediately and she carries on doing whatever she was doing before. She may even forget that she has asked that question as it disappears from her conscious awareness and it is replaced by other things. However, a little while later, maybe a few hours, days, or sometimes weeks later, an idea pops into her mind telling her where she knew the person she saw in the street from. How do you think this might happen?"

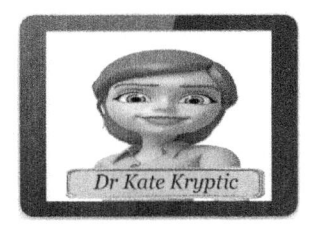

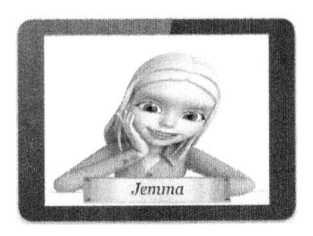

"Well I guess the little librarian had not forgotten that I asked that question, perhaps she was going through the filing cabinets looking for an answer or maybe she waited for me to go somewhere and suddenly remembered."

181

"That's what I'm saying. As soon as an opportunity occurred and there was space available on the whiteboard the librarian posted the information. A useful rule of thumb, therefore, will be to assume that when we ask our brain a question it will continue to work on questions posed to it even though we may have consciously forgotten that we have asked the questions in the first place."

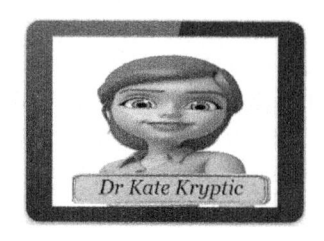

"Usually the little librarian will put thoughts or information in a queue to enter conscious awareness, and in this respect answers to questions you have asked will wait patiently to pop into your mind when there is space available or when the mind is not occupied with something else."

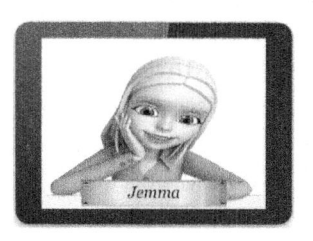

"Is that why so many thoughts go through my head at night just as I want to go to sleep?"

"Yes, that what I'm getting at. You will have access to these thoughts at night because your mind is not focussed on other things."

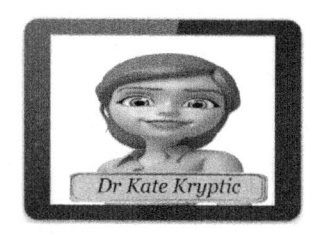

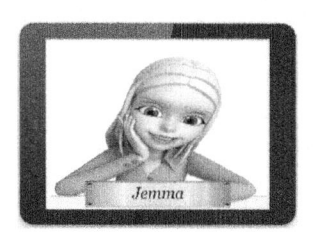

"What about the other thoughts you mentioned earlier. I think you said they were intrusive thoughts. I used to get those a lot?"

"Intrusive thoughts are different to the above mentioned patient type of thoughts that we have. They are not dissimilar to the librarian pushing through a registered letter for your attention. Intrusive thoughts are pushed through to consciousness, as a priority, pushing out any other information that is currently on line. You may be talking with someone when one of these thoughts pops into your head. For example, if you are socially anxious, an image of yourself looking odd could suddenly be pushed into your mind. Intrusive thoughts are sent with high degrees of importance and you will notice them as a result of the emotional intensity that comes with them."

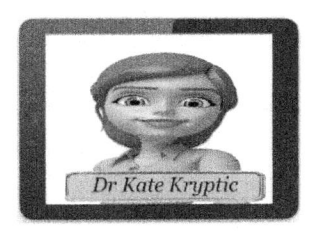

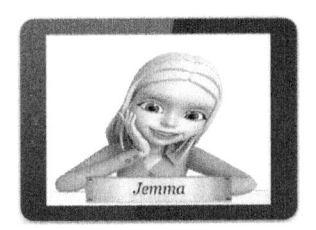

"So where do they come from?"

There may be many factors responsible for the creation of intrusive thoughts. One way that they may be generated is by worrying or asking "What if?" questions. This type of questioning process certainly appears to increase the likelihood of intrusive thoughts being pushed into consciousness. It is important to recognise than that when we receive intrusive thought messages they are not 'evidence' for anything. Although intrusive thoughts often feel uncomfortable, because they bring fear with them, it does not make these thoughts any more real than any other thoughts that pop into your mind."

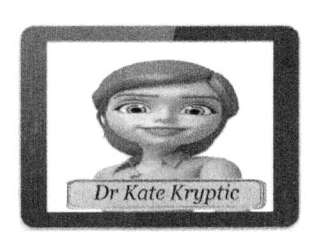

"I think the best way to explain this is by talking about a young man I worked with a little while ago."

"Gregory was a big worrier. He would often go through a process of worry, asking "What if?" questions to his mind and his brain would usually send him back the worst possible things that could happen, or what could go wrong. His intentions for worrying were positive as he felt that this type of questioning process could keep him safe. He thought that if he knew about the types of problems that might occur in advance then he could be prepared for them. Before going to the cinema with friends Gregory would ask himself about what could go wrong. His obedient mind usually sent him answers. One type of answer generated and sent to his conscious awareness was that he may end up in a middle seat feeling panicky, with everyone around noticing him, and he would feel humiliated."

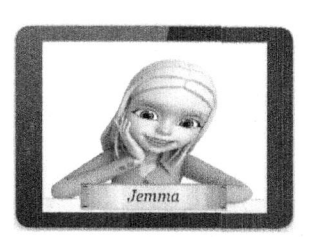

"I think most people would be anxious about that, wouldn't they?"

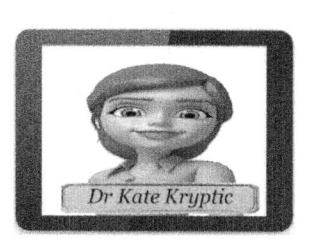

"The might do if they worried a lot about what people thought about them. But remember nothing had *actually* happened at this point. This was all in his mind. But, based on the ideas that his mind gave him Gregory decided to take action and sit at the back near an aisle seat so that he could make a quick exit if required. Gregory then began to think of how he could position himself in an aisle seat. He thought that if he could go in first in his group of friends he could stand near an aisle seat and gesture to others to go in ahead of him. His mind came up with a further ideas, such as if anyone questioned his need to sit in an aisle seat, he would say that he had a stomach ache and may need to go to the bathroom. He also had thoughts about phoning his friends up at the last minute and telling them that he couldn't make it. The amount of worrying that Gregory experienced before going to the cinema made the whole process of going to the cinema a difficult experience rather than the enjoyable experience that it could have been. Gregory's mind also reminded him how strange he was for engaging in this type of behaviour, and his friends would never think that he was like that."

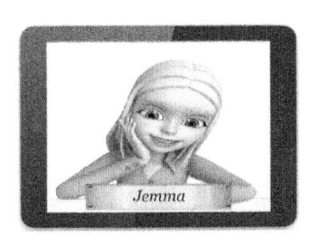

"So what happened to him?"

"A big risk for Gregory was deciding not to ask "What if?" questions. A big part of Gregory thought that asking himself these questions kept him prepared, safe and not vulnerable. Recognising that all thoughts that come into awareness are simply offerings sent by the mind and not ideas supported by evidence made a significant difference to Gregory. Gregory learnt how to stand back and observe his thoughts, and recognise that any thought that came into awareness was just a suggestion. Just because he had a thought did not mean it needed to be dealt with. As such, learning to notice his thoughts made a significant difference to him."

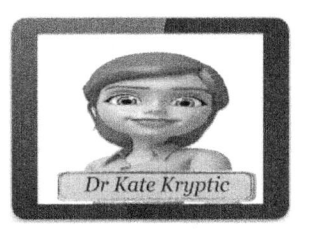

"Many people's minds come up with all sorts of negative ideas when they worry. In Gregory's case a worry for him was losing control, being thought of by others as weak, and others thinking that there was something wrong with him. I drew a diagram on my office white board for Gregory to look at. I have copied this onto the next page. It's same diagram that I mentioned earlier, that Christine Padesky uses."

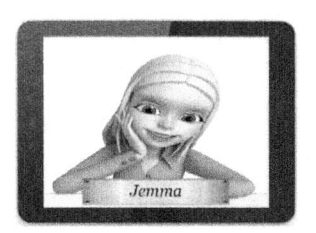

"Isn't she one of the authors of the book 'Mind Over Mood?"

"That right! Christine Padesky's ideas are very useful to us here to explain what was happening to Gregory. Gregory engaged in numerous avoidant type behaviours which tended to confirm his fear based thoughts still further. By carrying out avoidant behaviours Gregory did not collect alternative evidence that challenged his fears."

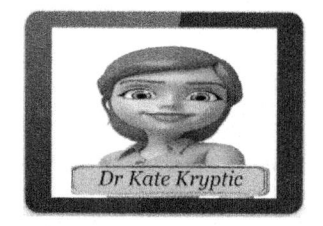

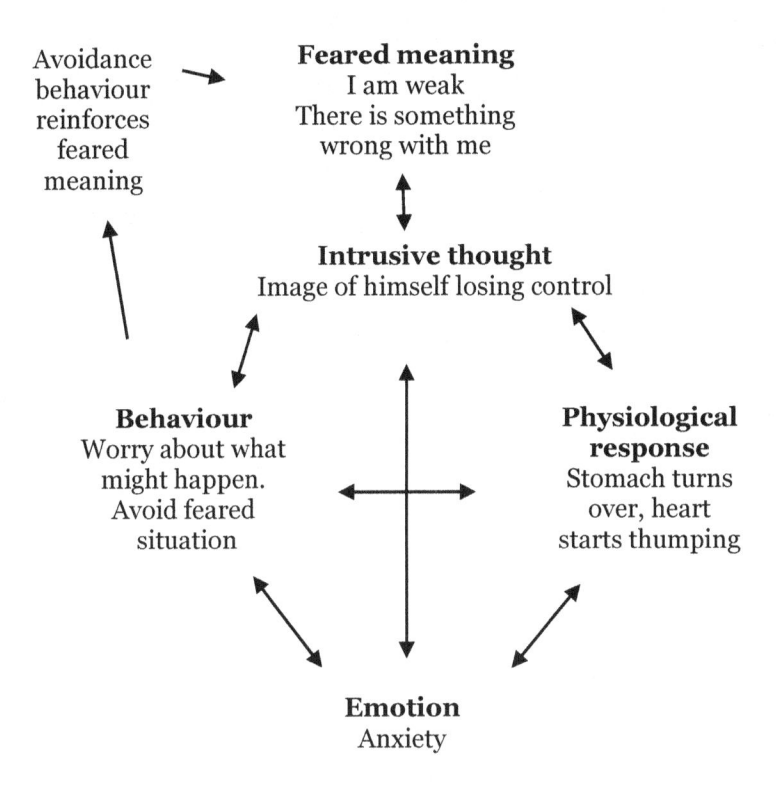

Avoidance behaviour reinforces feared meaning →

Feared meaning
I am weak
There is something wrong with me

↕

Intrusive thought
Image of himself losing control

Behaviour
Worry about what might happen. Avoid feared situation

Physiological response
Stomach turns over, heart starts thumping

Emotion
Anxiety

"The example on the previous page shows how the interactions between thoughts, feelings and behaviour have a tendency to maintain problems. In this case, interfering with Gregory's worry processes led to him having less frightening thoughts, which in turn led to a reduction in his tendency to want to avoid situations."

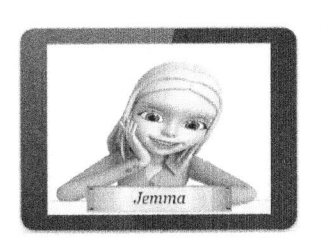

"So did that solve things for him?"

Jemma

"Unfortunately, we were not able to solve Gregory's problems by helping him to simply react to his thoughts in a different way, however. He also had several traumatic experiences from his past that we also needed to work through. Unless he confronted many of these fears there was the potential for him to continue to lead a more limited life than he needed to. We needed to work on these problems using more advanced methods of therapy."

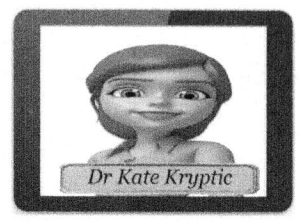

Dr Kate Kryptic

Chapter 17

Challenging safety behaviours

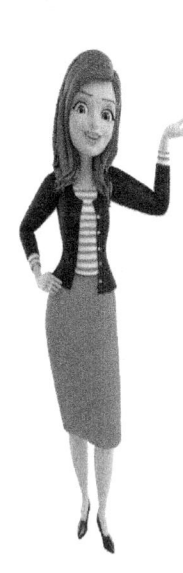

"In chapter 7 Kate made several lists of safety behaviours for people suffering with different conditions. Safety behaviours, work as part of a cycle that keeps problems in place for many people with mental health difficulties. As such, it is highly likely that your CBT therapist will talk to you about dropping them."

"Kate, what is the best way for our readers to approach doing something about their safety behaviours?

"Safety behaviours are often quite automatic and habitual so breaking them is not as easy as it might sound. The top part of the brain or the neo-cortex might recognise that in order to move on it will be necessary to drop safety behaviours. The bottom part of the mind or the primitive mind, however, will not want to let these safety behaviours go. The primitive mind learns best by experience rather than being told that something is OK."

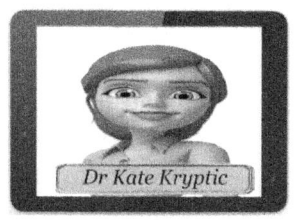

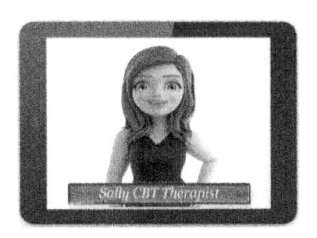

"So I guess our readers will need to somehow show the primitive parts of their minds that their safety behaviours don't work."

"Yes, that right Sally. With this in mind one of the most helpful ways to teach the primitive mind how to absorb new information is through experience. I will explain using an analogy."

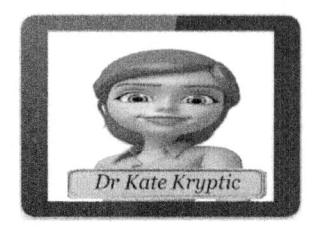

Dr Kate Kryptic

"I would like to invite you to think of the primitive mind as a child who comes to your bedroom door one night feeling frightened. You ask the child what she is frightened of and she says that she thinks there is something – a monster - in her wardrobe."

"You have several options in terms of your response. Your first set of responses could be to ignore, rationalise or avoid

- You could tell the child not to be so silly and completely <u>ignore</u> her. The result of this is that the child waits around outside your room and continues to try to gain your attention. She could even wait outside your bedroom door all night.
- You could <u>rationalise</u> with the child. You explain to her how impossible it is that a monster could get into her wardrobe and that monsters don't exist. You tell her that she is thinking about monsters because she watched a frightening television programme about monsters earlier. The result of this is that the child nods while listening and goes back to her room for a short while, but is back outside your room a few minutes later.
- You could <u>avoid</u> the problem by telling the child that she can sleep in a put-down bed in your room. The child is not scared anymore and happily gets into this bed. However, when the next day comes she seems more terrified than before of sleeping in her bedroom.

Or you could approach the problem

- You could take the child's hand acknowledging that she feels really frightened and tell her that you are both going to look into the wardrobe together. When you approach the wardrobe the child is really scared and she tries to resist going towards the wardrobe. You gently persist telling the child that it really is OK to feel frightened. When you have opened the wardrobe door and you both have had a good look inside for a couple of minutes you notice that the child has become a lot less anxious and is happier once more to sleep in her own bed. You don't hear any more from the child that night."

"With the last option you don't have to explain or rationalise, you simply help the child to acknowledge that she is scared. You take her to the situation which you know logically is very low risk. In other words you know there is a very low probability of there being a monster in her wardrobe. You then encourage her to find out for herself how dangerous the situation is. When this happens the child learns by her own experience. The primitive mind works in exactly the same way."

"There is one more thing to note in this area. The child looking in the wardrobe will need to do this without carrying out any ritualistic behaviours or safety mechanisms. Such behaviours could include crossing fingers, closing her eyes, holding onto a teddy bear etc. If the child uses these things for reassurance then the child will believe that her safety behaviours are keeping her safe and she will continue to need them. Remember many people who experience mental health problems and especially anxiety have safety behaviours, such as carrying diazepam, using beta-blockers, worrying, distracting the self by listening to music, being with a safe person and such like."

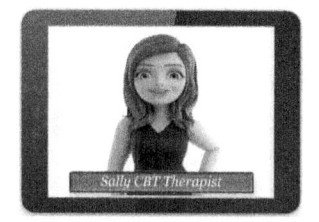

"So where do our readers start?"

"The best place for our readers to start will by **desensitising** themselves to their own fear reactions connected to dropping their safety behaviours. Desensitising means gradually being able to tolerate a feeling by staying in a situation until it feels more bearable."

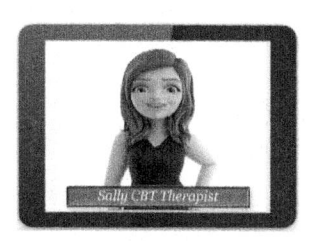

"What is the best way for our readers to do this?"

"To begin this our readers will need to bring into their awareness all of the safety behaviours that they currently fear dropping and all of the things that they have been avoiding. Many people will complete these types of lists with their therapist."

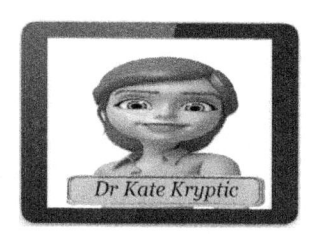

"One of the best places to start breaking down safety behaviours is to follow my recipe below."

1. Select a potential situation that produces relatively low levels of anxiety. For example, Vera in our previous chapter could ask to work in the village shop at a time when there are very few customers.
2. List all of the safety behaviours that you generally use in these types of situation. Many of these are listed in chapter 7.
3. For our readers benefit I have given an example list of safety behaviours in a table on the next page.
4. Rate every item on your list out of a maximum of 10 in terms of how anxious you think that they might feel if you were to drop this safety behaviour or to replace it with an alternative behaviour, for example, if our readers are suffering with social anxiety they could replace internal focus with external focus."
5. Start by dropping a safety behaviour that produces the lowest level of anxiety first and follow steps 6 to 10 below. You will then need to repeat the procedure repeatedly until your anxiety drops.
6. For each safety behaviour that you want to drop, describe what your new behaviour will be and how you will achieve it. I have put blank tables at the end of this chapter for our readers to use. Our readers can photocopy them if they wish.
7. Our readers will need to make a prediction about what they think might happen when they carry out an alternative behaviour.
8. Our readers will then need to try dropping their safety behaviour. Sometimes safety behaviours are easier to drop if they are replaced with another healthier behaviours.

9. Our readers will then need to use their table to write down what actually happened when they carried out their new behaviour.
10. Our readers can then think about what you learned from the process and share this with their therapist.
11. Finally our readers can then pick another safety behaviour with the next lowest level of anxiety associated with it and begin the process again.

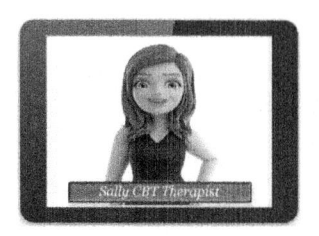

"I can see how this works in theory but how does this work in real life...I mean with clients?"

Sally CBT Therapist

"OK... This will be different according to what type of problem our reader is experiencing. Just for this example I will look at dropping safety behaviours in social anxiety. Jenny who was 16 had social anxiety and wanted to do things differently going forward. She wanted to practice dropping some of her safety behaviours and replacing them with other behaviours that she had discussed with her therapist. Two safety behaviours that Jenny chose to drop were self-monitoring and focusing internally. Jenny's completed CBT sheets are shown on the next pages. Jenny decided that initially she wanted to practice doing things differently with her cousin, who she trusted quite a lot, when she met her for a coffee.

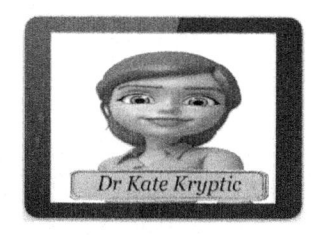

Dr Kate Kryptic

Jenny's safety behaviours and alternatives for social situations. Each situation is rated out of 10 with 10 being the highest level of fear.

Safety behaviour	Alternative behaviour (fear)
Spend excessive time preparing presentations for class	Reduce preparation time to the average taken by other students (10)
Rehearse answers in my mind before answering questions	Give answers to teachers speaking without thinking (9)
Focus on self to see how I am coming across	Focus on others instead of the self (External focus) (4)
Monitor self for signs of anxiety	Let anxiety be there (2)
Say as little as possible in social situations	Say what I think a bit more in social situations (6)
Stand in the background in social situations	Stand in a more prominent positions in social situations (3)
Arrive late for a social situation to minimise time spent socialising	Arrive earlier to a social event (5)
Worry beforehand about how I will cope with a social situation	Suspend worrying. Deal with difficulties only if or when a problem arises. (5)

Jenny's behavioural experiment sheet 1.

Safety behaviour : Monitor self for signs of anxiety
New behaviour (describe behaviour and how you will complete behaviour)
Drop monitoring. If I am aware that I am becoming anxious I will focus on accepting my anxiety and give it permission to be there.
Predictions about what will happen when you drop your safety behaviour. Write down as many scenarios as possible.
Probably nothing as my cousin knows me pretty well. My anxiety may surprise me and I could look awkward and say something silly or embarrassing.
What actually happened?
I became anxious at one point when there was a silence in the conversation. My stomach went over and I started to feel quite awkward. I focussed on allowing my anxiety to be there and my anxiety eased slightly. After a short while my cousin started talking about another subject.
What did I learn from this process?
My anxiety passed very quickly and my cousin did not seem concerned about it. Allowing anxiety to be there helps me feel slightly more relaxed.

Jenny's behavioural experiment sheet 2

Safety behaviour : Focus on myself to assess how I am coming across
New behaviour (describe behaviour and how you will complete behaviour)
Focus externally. I will place my attention as much as possible on my cousin and the environment. I will look at my cousin and listen to what she has to say.
Predictions about what will happen when you drop your safety behaviour. Write down as many scenarios as possible.
Looking at my cousin will make her feel uncomfortable and my anxiety will increase. I may feel less anxious as I will not be focussing on myself. I had a memory from the past of someone saying "What are you staring at?" and this sticks in my mind.
What actually happened?
I found that I felt much less anxious. At times I felt that I looking into myself but I pushed myself back into focusing externally.
What did I learn from this process?
It was much easier than I thought and I felt that I was much more relaxed. I am going to keep using this going forwards.

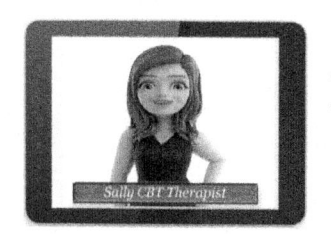

"Are there any other ways that our readers can work on reducing their safety behaviours?"

"One of the best ways for our readers to challenge their safety behaviours is by collecting their own evidence. A good way of achieving this is by repeatedly completing behavioural experiments in different situations, to collect information. At the end of this chapter I have put several examples of ways that our readers can challenge their safety behaviours. If our readers want to they can ask their therapist to work with them on dropping particular safety behaviours."

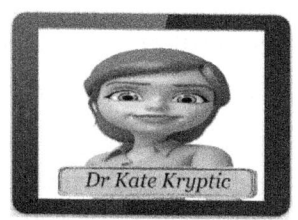

"As I mentioned earlier, once our readers become familiar with dropping safety behaviours, that are the easiest to drop they can then start to think about dropping behaviours that produce slightly more anxiety or discomfort. I have put Jenny's list of safety behaviours on the next page. It is very important that whenever our readers try new approaches that they accept their feelings while doing it. They will also need to be mindful that when they complete items on their list that they will need to do this without using any additional safety behaviours, such as holding their breath, distracting themselves and such like."

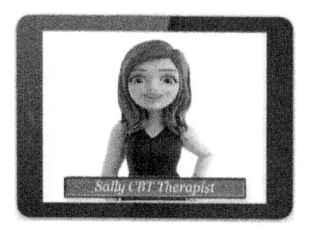

"And I guess that we will also need to remind our readers that it is not a good idea to move onto more challenging things until their anxiety about completing less challenging things has reduced significantly or is easily tolerated."

"That's right. Once they have practiced dropping their safety behaviours in situations where they have lower anxiety they can then progress through more difficult types of situations that they might generally avoid. For example, with Vera she could make things more challenging for herself by asking if she could work during a busy period at the shop. As with the exercises above, it is important that our readers do not move onto their more difficult challenges until their anxiety is reduced or very easy to tolerate. I have placed Jenny's social avoidance list below."

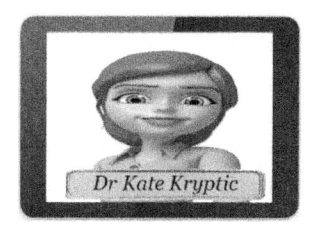

Jenny's social avoidance list

1. Meet cousin for coffee (2)
2. Have lunch with fellow students (4)
3. Agree to join a school committee (7)
4. Join a hockey club (7)
5. Attend a school get together (8)
6. Present to the class (9)
7. Join a debating society (10)
8. Go out on a date (10)

Potential behavioural experiments to discuss with your therapist if you are socially anxious

Safety behaviour	New alternative behaviour
Drink alcohol before going out to relax.	Go to social events in a state of sobriety.
Go to the toilet before going out (related to fear of using lavatories and others overhearing lavatory use.) Not being able to urinate at a urinal.	Use a lavatory in a public building. Use the lavatory while others are there. If male urinate in a urinal while other men are there. If unable to urinate wait for as long as is necessary.
Have someone with you when going to social situations.	Go to a social event alone.
Carry a bottle of water (to help with a dry mouth).	Leave water at home. Let dry mouth be there.
Sit close to an exit, so as to escape unnoticed.	Sit in a central area where you will have to move past people to leave the situation.
Hold onto or lean onto something supportive to hide shaking or trembling.	Allow hands to tremble. Allow others to see. Use external focus to assess what actually happens.
Wear light clothing, fan self or stand near a window or a doorway to prevent over-heating. Alternatively, wear more clothes to conceal sweating.	Wear normal clothing and stand in a warmer part of the room. Use external focus to assess what actually happens.

Potential behavioural experiments for social anxiety continued

Safety behaviour	New alternative behaviour
Have tissue ready to wipe hands to conceal sweaty hands.	Shake hands with somebody without wiping your hands first with tissues.
Use heavy makeup to avoid others noticing blushing or cover face with hair.	Use less make-up. Give permission for self to blush. Allow blushing experience to come and go. Use external focus to assess what actually happens.
Drink out a bottle rather than a glass to avoid others noticing shaking hands.	Drink out of a glass. If hands shake give permission for this to occur. Focus externally to assess what actually happens.
Have stories ready to put on an act of social competence and to have something interesting to say.	Go through a social event without telling stories or offering an acting performance. Practice active listening instead, using external focus.
Focus on self to assess social performance.	Focus on others. Be really curious and interested about what others think and how they behave.
Avoid conversations with people.	Start a conversation with a new person. Introduce yourself to them, by telling them your name.
Stand in a corner to keep a low profile.	Stand in a more prominent position where you are likely to interact with more people.

Safety behaviour	New alternative behaviour
Keep conversations as short as possible to avoid revealing anything that could be self-incriminating.	Offer up some information about yourself that you would not normally. Assess what others reactions are.
Focus on appearance.	Focus on what you like about other people's appearance.
Try to control facial expressions by focussing on face.	Focus externally and give permission for your face to do whatever it chooses.
Avoid eye-contact with others	Increase eye contact with others.
Mentally rehearse what is being said before it is said.	Speak without thinking and assess what actually happens.
Have excuses about why you need to leave pre-planned and ready.	Go to events without any pre-planning.

Potential behavioural experiments to discuss with your therapist if you have anxiety or panic attacks

Safety behaviour	New alternative behaviour
Carry a supply of supply of diazepam everywhere	Leave diazepam in the car when you visit the shops
Do not move too fast for fear of heart rate increase	Increase heart rate and observe what actually happens
Drink alcohol before going out to relax	Drink alcohol after you go out
Avoid situations where you have had panic attacks in the past	Gradually approach situations where panic attacks have occurred before
Do not eat before going out (if you have a fear of vomiting)	Eat a small meal before going out.
Go to the restroom before going out. If fear is related to loss of control of bowels	Hold off going to the restroom before going out unless you really need to go
Have a safe person with you	Leave safe person for a little while and see how you cope
Carry a brown paper bag to breath in and out of	Leave brown paper bag at home
Carry a bottle of water just in case of dry mouth	Hydrate with water before you go out.
Carry a plastic bag if fear is related to vomiting	Leave plastic bag at home for longer period
Sit near to an exit	Gradually sit further and further from an exit

Potential behavioural experiments to discuss with your therapist if you have anxiety or panic attacks

Safety behaviour	New alternative behaviour
Hold onto or lean onto something supportive	Trust your body's ability to balance without holding onto anything
Hold breath	Focus on breathing
Monitor anxiety	Focus externally
Fan self to stop self over heating	Give permission for body to heat up as much as it wants
Distract self to avoid noticing emotion	Focus on emotion, stay with it and take it with you

Potential behavioural experiments to discuss with your therapist if you are health anxious

Safety behaviour	New alternative behaviour
Monitor any unusual symptoms in body	Focus externally
Seek reassurance from loved ones	Hold off seeking reassurance
Make an appointment with Doctor	Limit appointments with doctor. Make appointment as far ahead as possible
Go onto the internet to complete research	Limit intent searched. Post phone internet searches
Complete on-line health assessments to self-diagnose	Watch television instead or read a book
Worry about ability to cope with various disorders	Decide to deal with eventualities if or when they happen
Request repeated medical tests from doctor	Limit tests to reasonable intervals discussed with your doctor
Request medical tests to rule out disorders when there are no symptoms	Wait for symptoms before requesting a medical test

Potential behavioural experiments to discuss with your therapist if you have obsessional compulsive disorder

Safety behaviour	New alternative behaviour
Avoid situations or people that may trigger obsessional thoughts	Carry out daily activities. Do not avoid people or places that you come across.
Retrace steps	Post phone retracing steps
Go back and check things that you are unsure of	If you have checked already once leave it.
Complete ritualistic behaviour, for example, touching wood.	Post ritualistic behaviour and wait for urge to die down
Complete mental calculations in head to distract from emotions	Put 100% attention onto feeling feelings
Push away intrusive thoughts. If you believe that thinking about them will make them real	Recognise intrusive thoughts. Allow them to come and go in their own time.
Complete activities a certain number of times	Reduce the number of time that you complete activities
Perform activities in a particular order	Deliberately change the order
Wear particular make-up or jewellery	Change make-up or jewellery
Carry certain items	Leave items behind for gradually longer periods of time
Check and re-check that you have not left anything behind	Check once and go

Potential behavioural experiments to discuss with your therapist if you have obsessional compulsive disorder

Safety behaviour	New alternative behaviour
Look for reassurance for others	Drop reassurance
Encourage others to engage in checks or rituals.	If you need to complete a checking behaviour do it on your own. Ask relatives not to co-operate with completing obsessional behaviours
Stay with safe people	Spend time away from safe people
Clean things to avoid contamination	Reduce cleaning activity. Post-phone cleaning.
Hold on items or hoard things	Gradually throw things that you don't need any more away. Thrown away a piece of unnecessary clutter at least once a day.

Potential behavioural experiments to discuss with your therapist if you have phobic anxiety

Safety behaviour	New alternative behaviour
Avoid particular objects or places	Gradually expose self to certain objects and places
Avoid certain forms of transport	Gradually approach transport. For example, enter stationary train. Get on and off. Work your way towards making a very small trip.
Take specific routes to avoid certain things such as bridges or motorways	Change route to approach feared things. For example, make a short journey on a quiet motorway, or travel across a small bridge
Avoid certain tastes, smells, sensations, feelings that might produce anxiety	Gradually learn to tolerate certain physical or sensory experiences
Ask for reassurance or others to check things for you.	Avoid asking for reassurance and if you need to check do it yourself
Avoid watching television about certain feared subjects	Watch programs about certain feared subjects. Make room for your feelings while you do this
Try to be in control of others. For example, if phobic of travel trying to give advice to the driver about how to drive safely	Allow others to drive.

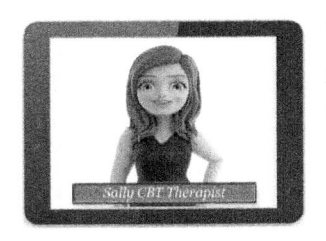

"I think completing behavioural experiments could be quite a challenge for our readers."

"Yes, it will be. Completing the above exercises can be very difficult, and many people find it easier to work through their lists with the help of a therapist. Most people find that their anxiety increases significantly when they challenge old ways of thinking and behaving. There does not need to be a timescale for dropping safety behaviours, but if our readers share what they are attempting to do with a trusted person this can be very helpful and can lead to reduced avoidance."

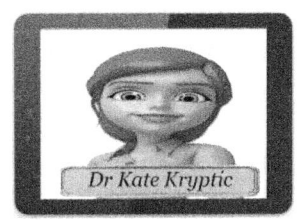

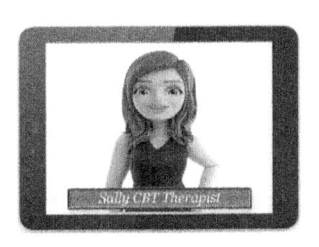

"Did you find that any of this happened to you Jemma?"

"Yes. It helped me telling my therapist what I was going to do. There was then kind of a pressure that I put on myself. I felt that I had to do it, because I knew she was going to ask me about it in my next session. Sometimes I didn't go through with things that I said I was going to do, and at first I was a bit nervous about telling her. But, in fact, my therapist was very nice about it. She helped me work out what was blocking me from doing things."

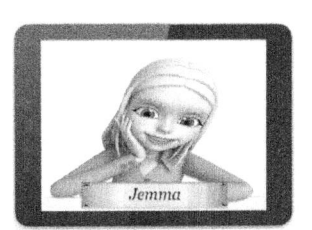

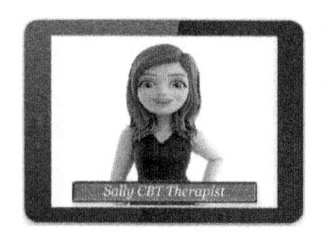

"Kate does this approach generally work for most people?"

"It works well for many people but not everyone. If our readers find that their anxiety does not reduce I would suggest that they don't carry on with this approach. It might be the case that there are unprocessed memories that need attention or working through. Unprocessed memories or traumas can often be an additional factor to anticipatory anxiety in the present time mode. Once unprocessed memories are worked through then it can be a lot easier to drop a safety behaviour afterwards.

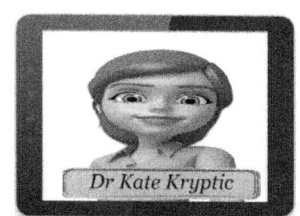

Chapter 17 – Further exploration

Systematic desensitisation sheets

Exposure work remains a large part of CBT. Perhaps the most effective way to approach feared situations or behaviours is to use a process known as systematic desensitisation. To complete systematic desensitisation you will need to write down a list of a) the things that you have been avoiding and b) behaviours that you fear carrying out. This list can be created in discussion with your therapist. Look at each item on your list and rate each item in terms of how much anxiety each item makes you feel.

To complete a systematic desensitisation process you will need to start with the least anxiety provoking item. Using the exposure worksheet in this chapter carry out the lowest anxiety provoking item until your anxiety reduces to zero or until your anxiety stabilises and you can easily tolerate your anxious feelings. It is important when you are carrying out systematic desensitisation that you **do not** move onto higher anxiety evoking items until you can easily tolerate lower anxiety evoking items. It is highly beneficial and good practice to repeat behaviours even when they feel mundane and/or boring. (For a full description of how to use these sheets please see the book CBT Worksheets).

Systematic desensitisation sheet

Feared situation or feared behaviour	What do I fear might happen?	Anxiety Rate out of 10 where 10 is the maximum

Behavioural experiment sheet

Describe old behaviour or safety behaviour

Describe new behaviour

How will you carry out new behaviour

Predictions about what will happen when you drop your safety behaviour. Write down as many scenarios as possible.

Carry out new behaviour and write down what actually happened here.

What did you learn from this process?
How likely are you to carry out this new behaviour again?

Exposure sheet

Time/date	Situation	Anxiety before (0 - 10 where 10 is max)	Anxiety during (0 - 10 where 10 is max)	Anxiety after (0 - 10 where 10 is max)	What did I learn?

Chapter 18

Conclusion

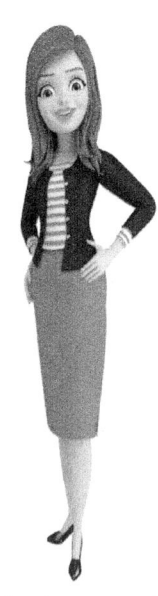

"We have now come to the end of our short introduction to CBT and how it works. There is a lot more to CBT than has been covered in this little book. If you like the style of writing in this book you could read in much more detail about your particular problems by reading our other books."

"In this book we covered some of the main areas that will be addressed in your CBT sessions. Now when you attend your CBT sessions hopefully you will have some idea of the types of things that will be discussed. In the back of this book I have placed some blank sheets that you can use before you have therapy if you wish."

"When you attend your assessment your therapist will ask you about what problems in particular you would like to work on. Picking a particular problem and writing down your thoughts and feelings about this problem will be very helpful, as you and your therapist will then be able to discuss it. You may also note down situations that lead to you feeling distressed, and how you think, feel and behave in these situations. The sheets at the back of this book will be helpful for making a record of what happens for you."

"If you are not sure what your main problems are you can complete our online questionnaire. This will give you an idea where you and your therapist might best focus your therapy.

http://www.z1b6.com/7.html

"You may also need to be aware before you start your CBT that it will involve you changing the way that you think, how you relate to your feelings and how you behave. Changing the way that you think, feel and behave is not as easy as it might seem, even if change is considered a good thing."

"Can you add anything about this Kate?"

"I certainly agree with you about fear of change Sally. Our readers are likely to meet resistance from themselves when they complete CBT, but if they can pass through this resistance they may learn new things from their new experiences and use what they learn in the future, hopefully even for the rest of their lives."

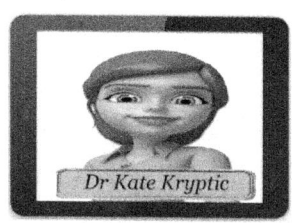

Dr Kate Kryptic

"After our readers have discussed their problems with their therapists they will have a much clearer idea about how their particular problem is being kept in place. Following this they will then be better placed to try out new coping strategies or different ways of thinking and behaving. They will be able to find out if making little changes here and there produces different results. I really hope our readers recognise how important it is that they give themselves the opportunity to try out alternative ideas when they have their CBT to assess what impact this has on the way they feel.

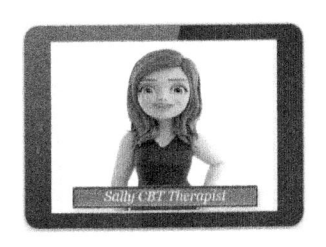

"How would this work practically in our reader's lives Kate?"

"To illustrate this I'd like you to imagine there's a fictional reader of this book called John Jones. Let's say that John has discussed his problems with his therapist and after his assessment realises what is keeping his problems in place. Based on what he learns in his therapy sessions John realises that many of the things that he was doing to reduce his distress were actually making his problems worse or keeping them in place."

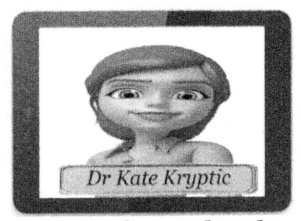

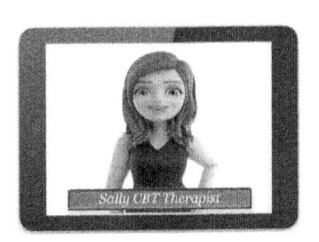

"So what happens next?"

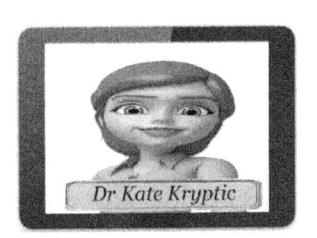

"Well, let's assume that John has a psychological explanation of what is happening to him, which he has worked out with his therapist. At first, however, John does not want to change his behaviour because it is unfamiliar to him. Eventually, he allows himself to get curious enough about what may occur if he behaves differently. After John does something differently for the first time, he then thinks to himself about the changes that he has noticed. This process of reflection helps John to cement his new approach in his mind which in turn encourages him to repeat similar approaches in the future."

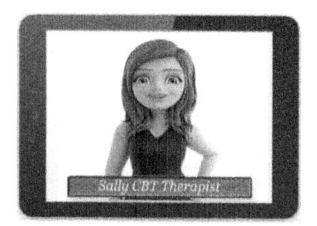

"So John fears change at first, does something new and then feels better about himself afterwards."

"Yes, that's what tends to happen. I would just like to let our readers know that if they notice that they want to resist change, this is completely natural. In my many years as a Clinical Psychologist, fear of change has cropped up frequently in my professional life. Embarrassingly, I will admit to you now Sally that I initially resist learning new therapeutic approaches thinking my current approach is the best way. I then approach the new therapy area and feel fear, anxiety and uncertainty while I learn to practice it. You see at this point these new approaches represent a challenge to my previous view of what I thought I knew, and I feel generally incompetent. I then gain the necessary knowledge about using the new approach, and my confidence in using it increases. The process then starts over again. Each time I do this I learn new things that can compliment and improve my understanding."

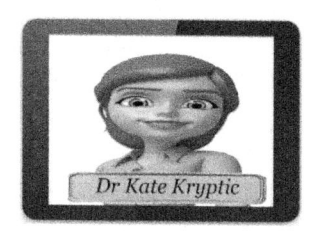

"So I guess what I'm saying is that although CBT will appear logical and scientific to our readers, carrying out the behaviour change that goes with it will be difficult for them."

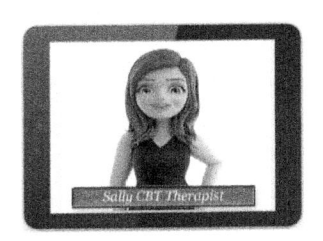

"What's you view on this Professor Knutt?"

"Much of it can be explained by the basal ganglia."

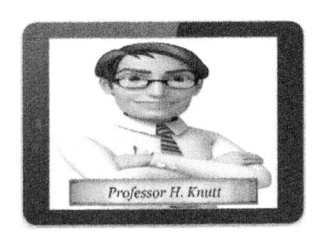

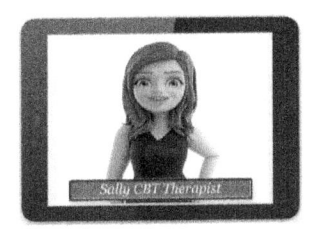

"That sounds intriguing. Please tell us more."

"OK, I mentioned this earlier but sometimes repetition is useful. Much of the time people can find themselves falling into repetitive loops or **habitual behaviours** when they become highly emotional. Habitual behaviours are behaviours that occur automatically. Many of us use the same habitual behaviours over and over again to deal with our emotions in certain situations, even when they our strategies don't work. Traditional neuroscience suggests that the seat of habit formation can be found in the basal ganglia, a sub-cortical region of the brain. I have placed a link below to a video about the basal ganglia, if our readers want to find out more about it."
http://www.z1b6.com/6.html

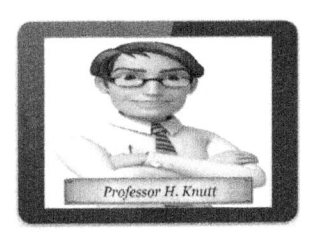

"When people are distressed, states of high emotional arousal lead to primitive brain areas located in the sub-cortical area taking a central role. These primitive brain areas are governed by habitual behaviour, which tends to be automatic, inflexible and rule-based. Habitual behaviour is generally thought to operate outside of conscious awareness and we revert to this quite strongly when under stress."

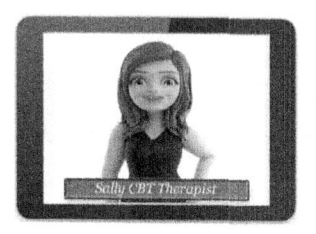

"So how does CBT help with habits stored in the basal ganglia?"

"CBT brings people's habitual behaviours to their awareness so that they can choose to do things differently. Breaking habitual cycles is not very easy because they are neurologically wired in. Once old cycles are broken, people can learn new positive habits. With repetition these new positive habits can then also be stored in the basal ganglia."

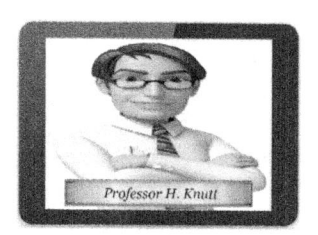

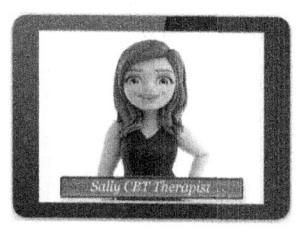

"Are there any other difficulties you think our readers might face when they complete CBT?"

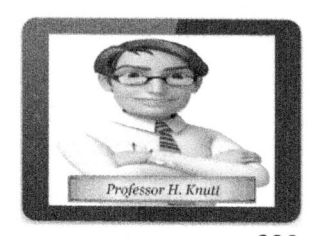

"Yes, like both Kate and Sally have already said, our readers might benefit by going into CBT expecting resistance to change from themselves every step of the way. We have a natural human tendency to resist change and to stay with what we know. Even when change is regarded as good, our natural human tendency is to put up resistance. I will illustrate the process for you below with an example. Hopefully our readers will note as they read on that changes in human thinking do not happen that readily."

"One thing that really frustrates me about science is that we continually fall into a habit of viewing theories or hypotheses as facts when in fact they are no more than a commonly held view."

"Let's imagine that in our past a common view was that the world was flat. This 'fact' 'the world is flat' was challenged by one scientist and he or she described an alternative worldview, in this case 'the world is round'. The scientist's new idea was supported by theoretical evidence, for example, the horizon had a slight curvature. The scientists' new suggestions met resistance from the general population as certainty was replaced by uncertainty, or as the previously stable view of the world was challenged. Suggestions were put forward to test the new theory, for example, someone said "Let's put a sailing expedition in place!" A guy called Magellan volunteered to complete the expedition and he set off to circumnavigate the world. Uncertainty, unrest, resistance and anxiety increased still further, as the challenge to the old worldview became **experiential**. Experiential means that we are experiencing things at a felt or real sense, not just thinking about things logically. The experiential phase of change is the most anxiety provoking for humans as it presents a position of "Not knowing." Potentially it is also one of the most frightening positions a thinking or conceptualising animal can find him or herself in, hence why we have such a built in avoidance of it. 'Not knowing' is associated with 'danger' and we are instinctively programmed to avoid what we perceive as dangerous."

"Eventually, Magellan comes back and the findings of his voyage are inspected and the results were measured. In this case the crew of the Magellan's expedition, brought back items from the other side of the world, drew new revised maps, and reported that the world was not flat. The previous view of the world had begun to change."

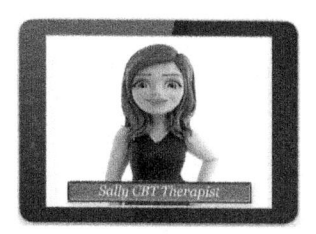

"So presumably things were finished there. Magellan had the evidence? The world was round!"

"Oh ... If only science were that easy! For a while there was still resistance, people disbelieved the evidence even though it was staring them in the face, and it was difficult for them to dispute it. However, after a period of time, uncertainty was gradually replaced by certainty and confidence in the new idea was reinforced. People's anxiety reduced and a period of reflection on the outcome followed. Eventually the new worldview was adopted by enough people, and it then became viewed as 'a fact.' After a while the whole process started again, when another scientist suggested that the world was not round it was a sphere flattened at its poles!"

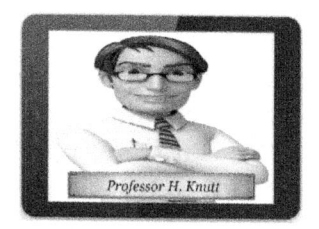

"I am suggesting that our readers' journey using a CBT model for particular problem will follow the same pattern in the same pre-determined order. A period of uncertainty will take place before change occurs. In this respect, as our readers approach the CBT interventions that they will come across in their therapy, periods of experiential uncertainty will become a natural and arguably essential part of their learning process. If they embrace this uncertainty or position of not knowing when they challenge their previously perceived view of the world they may also find that personal growth will be sidling up alongside them."

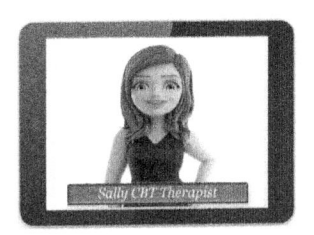

"So is that what you found when you had your therapy Jemma?"

"Definitely. I needed to find out what actually happened when I approached situations in a different way. As I mentioned earlier, my particular problem was social anxiety. For homework, I was given the task of trying a particular technique out when I went to visit my boyfriend's family. Even though I knew the exercise worked in sessions, because I'd already tried it with my therapist, I didn't want to try it out with my boyfriend's family. It felt too risky and I couldn't do it at first. It took me a few visits to my boyfriend's family before I actually did it. I gradually tried it more and more, and each time things were better. Now I use this particular technique most of the time."

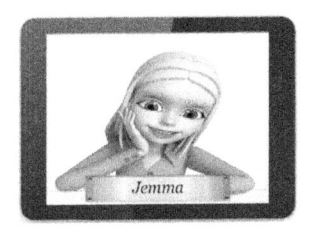

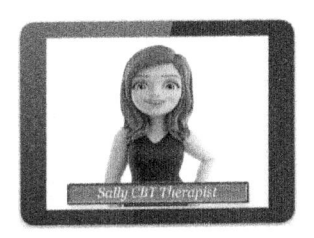

"So Kate what will happen if our readers embrace the uncertainty of completing their CBT?"

223

"As our readers progress with their therapy their uncertainty about the new exercises or new coping strategies completed will be replaced by increased certainty and confidence. Their distress will reduce and they will begin to reflect on the outcomes that they have achieved. The process will then begin again with the next new exercise that they try."

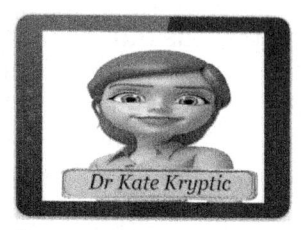

    ... Very best of luck with your therapy ....

Index
Academics, 22
Amygdala, 29, 40, 47, 116
Basal Ganglia, 29, 35, 36, 172, 219, 220
Behavioural experiments, 196-209
Behavioural strategies, 149
Catecholamines, 41-47
Cognitive distortions, 95, 98
Cognitive interventions, 149-150
Consciousness, 15, 48, 65, 175, 179, 182-184
Coping strategies, 15
Core beliefs, 126
Counter-intuitive, 126, 165
Depression, 57 -79, 105, 136, 153
Desensitising, 192, 211
Diazepam, 78, 80, 192, 203
Downward arrow, 118-119, 127, 127
Experiential, 221, 225
External focus, 193, 195, 200, 201
Fight-flight, 40, 47, 51
Goals, 139
Habitual behaviours, 35-36, 172, 219-220
Health anxiety, 37, 81, 138, 149, 153
Hippocampus, 64, 86
Holistic, 33
Holocaust, 117
Hypothesis, 105, 221
Interpretative bias, 69,
Intrusive thoughts, 175, 183, 184, 206
LeDoux, 53
Limbic system, 29-30
Limiting beliefs, 113-118, 125
Maladaptive, 107
Magellan, 221-222
Mindfulness, 64-65
Mood regulation, 85
Negative automatic thoughts, 152, 155
Negative reinforcement, 74

Index (continued)

Neo-cortex, 28-30, 44, 46, 48, 52, 68, 166, 189
Obsessional compulsive disorder, 81-82, 206-207
Padesky, 135, 157-159, 186-187
Panic attacks, 50, 54, 80, 203, 204
Phobic anxiety, 51, 82, 208-209
Phobic response, 51
Plasticity, 64, 86
Post-traumatic stress disorder, 82
Pre-frontal cortex, 29, 30, 43, 44, 46, 48, 64, 69, 85-87
Registered therapists, 23
Rules, 101-109, 125-126, 130
Rumination, 64, 69, 173, 175
Safety behaviours, 71-78, 113, 130, 162, 189, 191-195, 198-199
Self-observation, 83, 87
Serotonin, 65-68
Serotonin re-uptake inhibitors, 65-68
Social anxiety, 78, 79, 138, 153, 155, 159, 193, 194, 201
Subcortical regions, 29-36, 40, 46, 51-53, 86, 166, 172, 220
Thought challenging, 155, 158
Tryptophan, 67
Unprocessed memories, 51-54, 210
Worry, 47, 48, 74, 81, 106, 167, 173-175, 184-187, 192, 211, 195, 205

Regulatory organisations in the UK

British Association of Cognitive and Behavioural Psychotherapists
Imperial House
Hornby Street
Bury
Lancashire
BL9 5BN
Tel: 0161 705 4304   Fax: 0161 705 4306
Email: **babcp@babcp.com**

British Association for Counselling & Psychotherapy
BACP House
15 St John's Business Park
Lutterworth
LE17 4HB
Tel 01455 883300

British Psychological Society
St Andrews House
48 Princess Road East
Leicester
LE1 7DR
United Kingdom
Tel: +44 (0)116 254 9568
Fax: +44 (0)116 227 1314
Email: **enquiries@bps.org.uk**

Health & Care Professional Council
Park House
184 Kennington Park Road,
London
SE11 4BU,
0300 500 6184

Glossary of terms

Academics - Academics spend a lot of time studying or researching specialist subjects at institutions like universities.

Abdominal breathing – Processing of breathing which involves relaxing the abdomen and taking in air to the bottom of the lungs.

Amygdala – Small area of brain tissue within the limbic system, responsible for activating the body's fight-flight-or-freeze response.

Anxiety – An emotion which is experienced when the body is moving into a prepared state to deal with a potential threat.

Automatic responses – Responses which occur automatically/outside of conscious awareness.

Behavioural strategies – Making an adjustment to your behaviour and monitoring the impact of resulting changes.

Catastrophic misinterpretation – A frightening and exaggerated thought connected to magnification of perceived stimuli.

Catecholamines – Chemical messengers used by cells to communicate with one and other.

Cognitive distortions – Thinking patterns that distort perception of reality.

Cognitive models – Ways of explaining how psychological distress is maintained.

Cognitive interventions – Strategies based on changing mental reactions.

Conditioned response – A response that occurs automatically as a result of repeated actions towards particular stimuli.

Coping strategies – Strategies that have been of some assistance in reducing distress.

Core beliefs – Strongly held beliefs about the self.

Counter-intuitive – Ideas which we would not naturally gravitate towards.

Default response – An automatic response based on previous experiences and past conditioning.

Desensitising - Gradually being able to tolerate a feeling by staying in a situation until the feeling feels more bearable.

Diazepam – A medication often prescribed as a muscle relaxant.

Dissociation – A mental and physical state where an individual feels a loss of connection with his or her body.

Distraction – A process that individuals use to avoid experiencing painful emotions.

Emotional reference point – A mechanism used by babies who look towards caregivers to determine how they might react at an emotional level.

Experiential – A process of experiencing through the senses.

External focus – Placing one's attention onto ones external environment.

Habitual behaviours – Behaviours that we are inclined to do because we have do because we have done them so many times before.

Holistic – Multiple process connected together working in parallel.

Hyperventilation – A process of rapid shallow breathing where an individual breathes out too much carbon dioxide.

Hypothesis – An idea based on scientific theory.

Intrusive thoughts – Thoughts that enter awareness uninvited. These thought are usually accompanied by heightened emotion.

Mindfulness – A process of staying in the present moment, bringing conscious awareness back to the present, and deliberately moving away from thoughts about the past or the future.

Mood regulation – An ability to have some management of one's feelings.

Negative automatic thoughts - Thoughts in the background of the mind that have the potential to keep individuals emotionally distressed.

Negative reinforcement – A process of repeated behaviour in which negative emotion is reduced leading to greater likelihood of the same future behaviour.

Neo-cortex – Highly developed area of the mind responsible for logical, rational and analytical thinking.

Phobic response – An automatic response associated with heightened anxiety, connected to a specific trigger or cue.

Plasticity – The brains ability to repair itself and grow the more that it is used.

Prefrontal cortex – An area of the brain that acts as a relay between the subcortical regions of the brain and the neo-cortex. It is also responsible for dampening emotional reactions and quietening the mind.

Registered therapists – Registered therapists are members of professional bodies. Professional bodies are organisations that check out their therapists to make sure that they have the required training to do their jobs properly.

Rumination – A cognitive process which involves churning of thoughts connected to the self in the past over and over in the mind.

Safety behaviours - Behaviours utilised to reduce emotional distress in the short-term.

Self-fulfilling prophesy – When something occurs despite your very best attempts to prevent that particular thing occurring.

Self-perpetuating – A situation that is kept in place through its own actions.

Serotonin - A chemical messenger serotine plays a huge part in the body's overall physical and mental Functioning.

Subcortical regions – Brain areas located in the lower half of the brain.

Supressing emotions – An act of pushing down painful or upsetting feelings.

Threat Perception Centre – An area within the brain responsible to noticing stimuli associated with past fear or trauma.

Traumatic incidents – Events that have occurred in the past connected to highly distressing emotions.
Unprocessed memory - An experience that the mind has not fully dealt with.

Vicarious trauma - When people develop trauma responses as a result of observing other people's intense emotional reactions.

References

Arnsten, A, Raskind, M. Taylor, F, & Connor, D. *Neurobiology of Stress* (2015). The effects of stress exposure on prefrontal cortex: Translating basic research into successful treatments for post-traumatic stress disorder, pages 89–99

Bandura, A., (1977). *Social Learning Theory*. Prentice-Hall.

Beck, J. (2011) *Cognitive Behavior Therapy: Second Edition – Basics and Beyond*. The Guildford Press.

Butler, G., (2009). *Overcoming Social Anxiety & Shyness*. Robinson

Clark, D.M., (1986) A cognitive approach to panic: *Behaviour Research and Therapy*, 24: 461-470

Cabral, R & Nardi E. *(2012)*. Anxiety and inhibition of panic attacks within translational and prospective research contexts. *Trends in Psychiatry*

Debiec J., & Sullivan, R. (2014). Intergenerational transmission of emotional trauma through amygdala-dependent mother-to-infant transfer of specific fear. *PNAS*, DOI: 10.1073/pnas.1316740111

Golman, D., (1996) .Emotional intelligence: Why it can matter more than IQ. Bloomsbury

Guzmán, Y., Tronson, N., Jovasevic, K., Sato, K., Guedea, A., Mizukami, H., Nishimori, K., & Radulovic. J. (2013) Fear-enhancing effects of septal oxytocin receptors. *Nature Neuroscience*, 2013; DOI: 10.1038/nn.3465

Greenberger, D., & Padesky, C. (1995). *Mind Over Mood: Change How You Feel by Changing the Way That You Think*. Guildford Press Kennerley, H., (2009).
Kennerley, H., (2009). *Overcoming anxiety: A self-help guide using cognitive behavioural techniques*. Robinson

Kinman, G & Grant, L. (2010). Exploring Stress Resilience in Trainee Social Workers: The Role of Emotional and Social Competencies. *British Journal of Social Work*. 10.1093/bjsw/bcq088

Krusemark, E & Li. W., (2012). Enhanced Olfactory Sensory Perception of Threat in Anxiety: An Event-Related fMRI Study (2012). *Chemosensory Perception*, 5 (1): 37 DOI: 10.1007/s12078-011-9111-7

LeDoux JE[1], Iwata J, Cicchetti P, Reis DJ. Different projections of the central amygdaloid nucleus mediate autonomic and behavioral correlates of conditioned fear (1988). *J Neurosci.* Jul;8(7):2517-29.

Logue, M.W., Bauver, S.R., Kremen, W.S., Franz, C.E., Eisen, S.A., Tsuang, M.T., Grant, MD., & Lyons, M.J., (2011). Evidence of Overlapping Genetic Diathesis of Panic Attacks and Gastrointestinal Disorders in a Sample of Male Twin (2011).*Twin Res Hum Genet*. Feb; 14(1): 16–24. doi: 10.1375/twin.14.1.16

McIlrath, D & Huitt, W. The teaching-learning process: A discussion of models. *Educational Psychology Interactive*. Valdosta, GA: Valdosta State University. Retrieved 2016 from http://www.edpsycinteractive.org/papers/modeltch.html

Moulding, Richard, Coles, Meredith E., Abramowitz, Jonathan S., Alcolado,Gillian M., Alonso, Pino, Belloch, Amparo, Bouvard, Martine, Clark, David A., Doron, Guy, Fernández-Álvarez, Hector, García-Soriano, Gemma, Ghisi, Marta, Gómez, Beatriz, Inozu, Mujgan, Radomsky, Adam S., Shams, Giti, Sica, Claudio, Simos, Gregoris & Wong, Wing (2014). Part 2. They scare because we care: the relationship between obsessive intrusive thoughts and appraisals and control strategies across 15 cities., *Journal of obsessive-compulsive and related disorders*, vol. 3, no. 3, pp. 280-291.

Rachman, S., Coughtrey, Shafran, R & Radomsky, A., (2015). *The Oxford Guide to the Treatment of Mental Contamination*. The Oxford University Press

Teachman, B., Marker, C & Clerkin, E. (2010). Catastrophic misinterpretations as a predictor of symptom change during treatment for panic disorder (2010). *Consult Clin Psychol*. 78(6): 964–973.

Veale, D., & Wilson, R., (2005). *Overcoming Obsessive Compulsive Disorder: A self-help guide using Cognitive Behavioral Techniques*.. Constable & Robinson Ltd

Wells, A. (1997) Cognitive Therapy of Anxiety Disorders: A Practice Manual and Conceptual Guide. Wiley.

Common medications prescribed for anxiety disorders or for anxiety disorders with co-morbid depression

Alprazolam – A benzodiazepine prescribed for panic, generalised anxiety, phobias, social anxiety, OCD

Amitriptyline – A tricyclic antidepressant

Atenolol – A beta-blocker prescribed for anxiety

Buspirone – A mild tranquiliser prescribed for generalised anxiety, OCD and panic

Chlordiazepoxide – A benzodiazepine prescribed for generalised anxiety, phobias

Citalopram – A selective serotonin reuptake inhibitor commonly prescribed for mixed anxiety and depression

Clomipramine – A tricyclic antidepressant

Clonazepam – A benzodiazepine prescribed for panic, generalised anxiety, phobias, social anxiety

Desipramine – A tricyclic anti-depressant

Diazepam – A benzodiazepine prescribed for generalised anxiety, panic, phobias

Doxepin – A tricyclic antidepressant
Duloxetine – A serotonin-norepinephrine reuptake inhibitor

Escitalopram Oxalate – A selective serotonin reuptake inhibitor

Fluoxetine - A selective serotonin reuptake inhibitor

Fluvoxamine – A selective serotonin reuptake inhibitor

Gabapentin – An anticonvulsant prescribed for generalised anxiety and social anxiety

Imipramine – A tri-cyclic antidepressant

Lorazepam – A benzodiazepine prescribed for generalised anxiety, panic, phobias

Nortriptyline – A tricyclic antidepressant

Oxazepam – A benzodiazepine prescribed for generalised anxiety, phobias

Paroxetine – A selective serotonin reuptake inhibitor

Phenelzine – A monoamine oxidase inhibitor

Pregabalin – An anticonvulsant prescribed for generalised anxiety disorder

Propanalol – A beta blocker prescribed for anxiety

Sertraline - A selective serotonin reuptake inhibitor

Tranylcypromine – A monoamine oxidase inhibitor

Valproate – An anti-convulsant prescribed for panic

Venlafaxine – A serotonin-norepinephrine reuptake inhibitor

Additional worksheets (from the book CBT Worksheets, by Dr James Manning & Dr Nicola Ridgeway)

Therapy preparation sheet

Describe problem I have been experiencing?

How long has this problem been around for?

What may have triggered my problem?

How have I attempted to resolve my problem?

What are the main things that keep my problem in place?

What will I need to do to resolve this problem?

How would my life be different without this problem?

Activity schedule

Time	Monday			Tuesday			Wednesday			Thursday			Friday			Saturday			Sunday		
	Activity	H	A	Activity	H	A	Activity	H	A	Activity	H	A	Activity	H	A	Activity	H	A	Activity	H	A
8.00 am to 9.00 am																					
9.00 am to 10.00 am																					
10.00 am to 11.00 am																					
11.00 am to 12.00 pm																					
12.00 pm to 1.00 pm																					
1.00 pm to 2.00 pm																					
2.00 pm to 3.00 pm																					
3.00 pm to 4.00 pm																					
4.00 pm to 5.00 pm																					
5.00 pm to 6.00 pm																					
6.00 pm to 7.00 pm																					
7.00 pm to 8.00 pm																					

Write down the main thing that you are doing in each hour time period.

After you have completed the activity score yourself in terms of achievement and happiness giving yourself a score between 0 and 10, where 10 is the highest it can possibly be and 10 is the lowest.

H = Happiness
A = Achievement

Anger diary

Time Date	Trigger	Thoughts	Emotion	Bodily changes	Behaviour	Consequences of behaviour

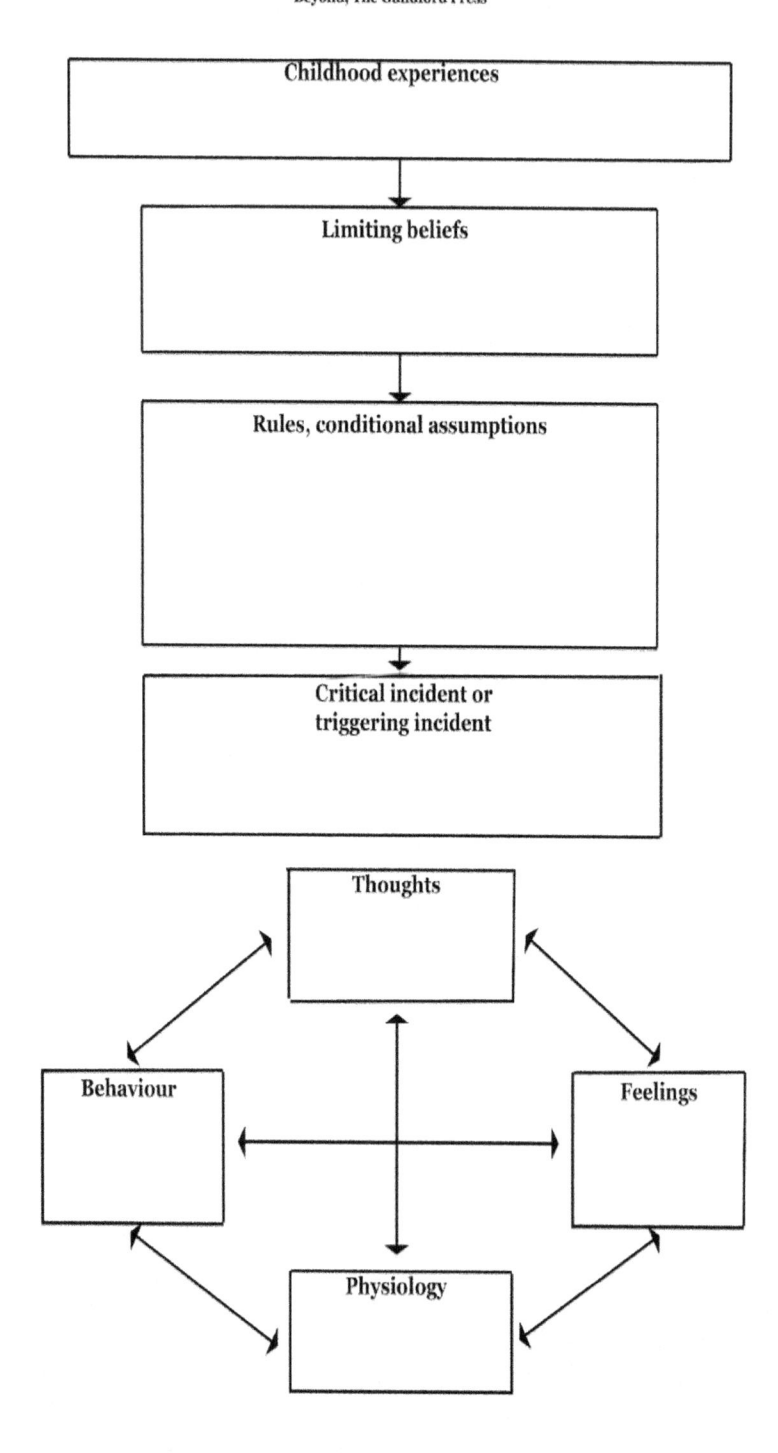

Longitudinal CBT Model based on Judith Beck. Beck, J. (2011). Cognitive therapy: Basics and Beyond; The Guildford Press

```
┌─────────────────────────────┐
│   Childhood experiences     │
└──────────────┬──────────────┘
               ↓
┌─────────────────────────────┐
│     Limiting beliefs        │
└──────────────┬──────────────┘
               ↓
┌─────────────────────────────┐
│  Rules, conditional         │
│  assumptions                │
└──────────────┬──────────────┘
               ↓
┌─────────────────────────────┐
│  Critical incident or       │
│  triggering incident        │
└─────────────────────────────┘
```

```
              Thoughts
             ↗   ↕   ↖
            ↙         ↘
     Behaviour ←→ ←→ Feelings
            ↖         ↗
             ↘   ↕   ↙
             Physiology
```

Responsibility Pie

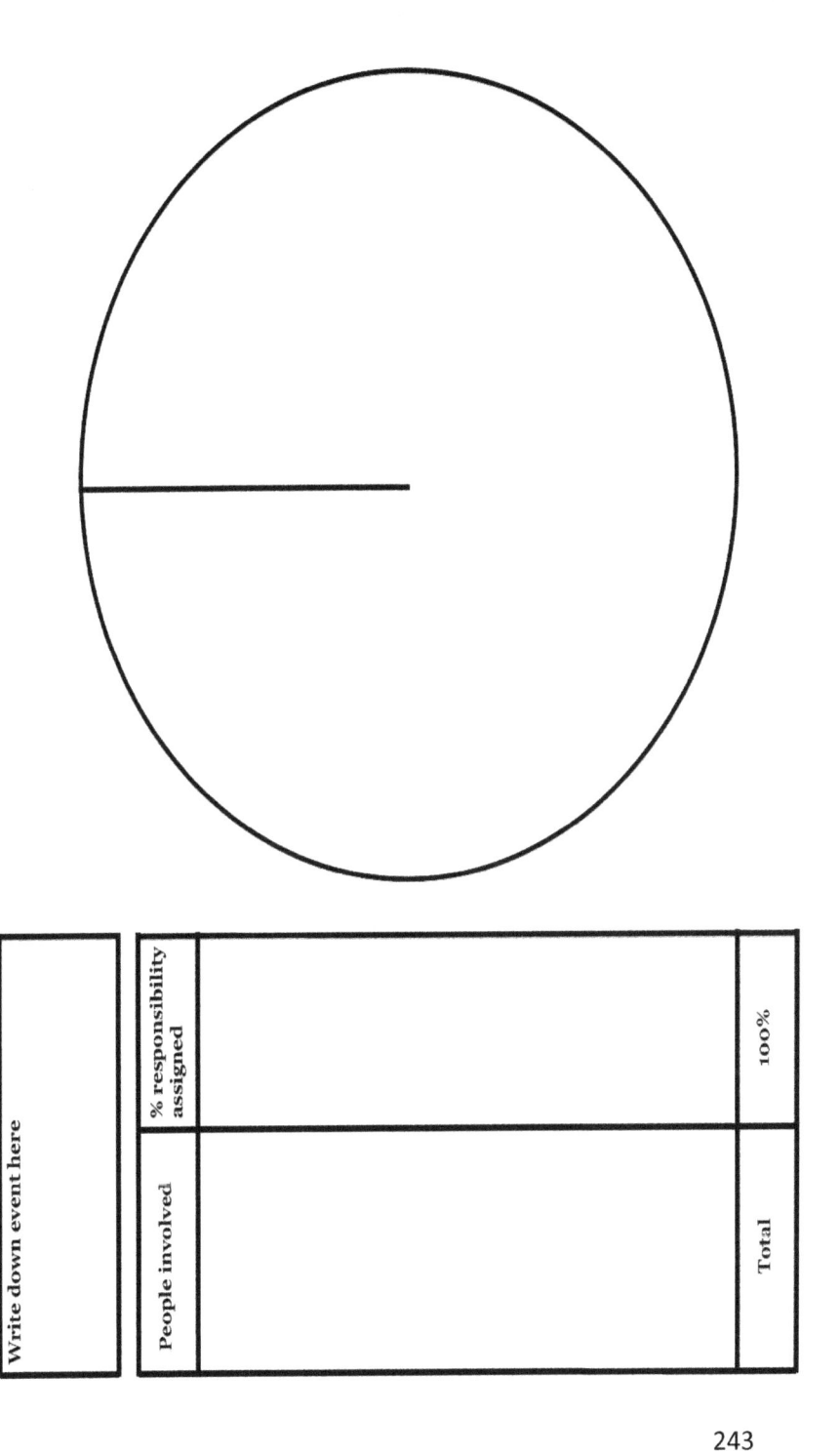

Write down event here		
People involved	% responsibility assigned	
Total	100%	

243

There now follow an extract from

The Little Book on CBT for Depression

By Dr Nicola Ridgeway. ClinPsyd & Dr James Manning, ClinPsyD

SESSION 3 - THOUGHTS THAT DON'T REFLECT REALITY

CONSCIOUSNESS IS STILL NOT FULLY UNDERSTOOD, AND EVIDENCE INDICATES THAT SOME PARTS OF THE BRAIN DO NOT UNDERSTAND THE DIFFERENCE BETWEEN REALITY AND FICTION

CLIENT: Well ... my brain definitely understands the difference

THERAPIST: I wonder if we might consider an illustration of this point?

Just for a moment close your eyes.

Now, imagine that you have a tray on your lap. Now, just imagine that there is a lemon on the tray. Next to the lemon there is a fruit knife. Look at the lemon, and pay careful attention to its texture, colour and smell. Pay attention to the shape of the lemon. Now, reach out and place one hand on the knife. Just be aware of how the lemon juice runs on your fingers ... and now, very carefully, pick up a small piece of lemon and slowly bring it towards your mouth ... and just place it on your tongue ... and when you've done that , open your eyes and bring your awareness back to where you are. So what did you notice when you brought the lemon to your lips?

CLIENT: My mouth started to salivate.

THERAPIST: Brilliant! What do you make of the idea that your mouth had a reaction to the lemon, even though there was no lemon there? How could that be?

CLIENT: That's weird ... I guess I must have made it happen because I imagined it as if it was happening.

THERAPIST: Yes, exactly! You experienced that reaction because you expected it. What might that tell you about the power of your thoughts?

CLIENT: That my thoughts can have a very powerful impact on my body.

THERAPIST: This is the same for a lot of our thought processes. As soon as we think of an event, parts of our brain begin to activate a physiological response to it as if it were real.

CLIENT: So what you're saying is ... if I dwell on negative things happening in my life, I'll start to feel depressed.

THERAPIST: Exactly! When we think about or visualise painful events our bodies create a parallel physiological reaction matching the thought. This is why thinking about painful thoughts can bring about very intense feelings.

Lightning Source UK Ltd.
Milton Keynes UK
UKOW05f1922271016
286331UK00019B/1050/P